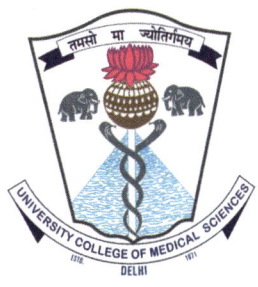

University College of Medical Sciences

Dilshad Garden, Delhi

Microbiology
Practical Manual

Department of Microbiology

Student Particulars

Name _____

Roll No. _____   Year/Session _____

University Roll No. _____   Name of the Course _____

This is to certify that this is a bonafide practical work done by _____
during the year 20____ – 20____. His/her work is complete | incomplete | excellent | satisfactory | good | fair.

_____   _____
Signature of Staff In-charge   Signature of Professor & HoD

Submitted for University Examination in the year _____

Examiners: _____   _____

Microbiology
Practical Manual

Rumpa Saha MBBS MD

Professor
Department of Microbiology
University College of Medical Sciences and GTBH
Dilshad Garden, Delhi

Shukla Das MBBS MD DNB MNAMS

Director-Professor
Department of Microbiology
University College of Medical Sciences and GTBH
Dilshad Garden, Delhi

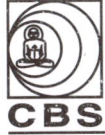
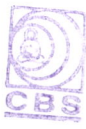

CBS Publishers & Distributors Pvt Ltd

New Delhi • Bengaluru • Chennai • Kochi • Kolkata • Mumbai

Bhopal • Bhubaneswar • Hyderabad • Jharkhand • Nagpur • Patna • Pune • Uttarakhand • Dhaka (Bangladesh) • Kathmandu (Nepal)

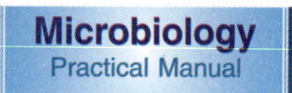

ISBN: 978-81-94125-45-7

Copyright © Authors and Publisher

First Edition: 2020

Published by Satish Kumar Jain and produced by Varun Jain for

CBS Publishers & Distributors Pvt Ltd

4819/XI Prahlad Street, 24 Ansari Road, Daryaganj, New Delhi 110 002, India.
Ph: 011-23289259, 23266861, 23266867   Fax: 011-23243014   Website: www.cbspd.com
                                                                e-mail: delhi@cbspd.com; cbspubs@airtelmail.in

Corporate Office: 204 FIE, Industrial Area, Patparganj, Delhi 110 092
Ph: 011-49344934   Fax: 011-49344935   e-mail: publishing@cbspd.com; publicity@cbspd.com

Branches

- **Bengaluru:** Seema House 2975, 17th Cross, K.R. Road,
  Banasankari 2nd Stage, Bengaluru 560 070, Karnataka
  Ph: +91-80-26771678/79   Fax: +91-80-26771680   e-mail: bangalore@cbspd.com
- **Chennai:** 7, Subbaraya Street, Shenoy Nagar, Chennai 600 030, Tamil Nadu
  Ph: +91-44-26680620, 26681266   Fax: +91-44-42032115   e-mail: chennai@cbspd.com
- **Kochi:** 42/1325, 1326, Power House Road, Opposite KSEB Power House,
  Ernakulam 682 018, Kochi, Kerala
  Ph: +91-484-4059061-65   Fax: +91-484-4059065   e-mail: kochi@cbspd.com
- **Kolkata:** 6/B, Ground Floor, Rameswar Shaw Road, Kolkata-700 014, West Bengal
  Ph: +91-33-22891126, 22891127, 22891128   e-mail: kolkata@cbspd.com
- **Mumbai:** 83-C, Dr E Moses Road, Worli, Mumbai-400018, Maharashtra
  Ph: +91-22-24902340/41   Fax: +91-22-24902342   e-mail: mumbai@cbspd.com

Representatives

- **Bhopal**   0-8319310552
- **Jharkhand**   0-9811541605
- **Pune**   0-9623451994
- **Kathmandu**   977-9818742655
  (Nepal)

- **Bhubaneswar**   0-9911037372
- **Nagpur**   0-9421945513
- **Uttarakhand**   0-9716462459

- **Hyderabad**   0-9885175004
- **Patna**   0-9334159340
- **Dhaka (Bangladesh)** 01912-003485

Printed At : Goyal Offset Works (P) Limited

Foreword

The existence of microorganism was predicted many centuries ago in Jain's literature and by Marcus Terentous Varro in ancient Rome. Louis Pasteur and Robert Koch are the founders of medical microbiology. The life expectancy has increased many folds over last 100 years after the development of microbiological techniques. The understanding of microorganisms and microbiological techniques plays an important role for MBBS students in learning the biological basis of disease and its remedies. The learning process has to be gradual, stepwise and crystal clear.

It gives me great privilege to write the Foreword of the book *Microbiology Practical Manual*.

The authors are well known to me for more than a decade and are very motivated and ambitious. They are very experienced in teaching microbiology and are well versed in conducting undergraduate examinations for MBBS students. I have observed keenness and steady craving in them to learn more and endeavour towards perfection. Their eagerness to impart the sound education and create a clinician with clear understanding of the subject is being reflected in developing this manual.

This manual is structured to cover all the practical techniques of microbiology as is being taught and shown to them to achieve uniformity in learning. Hence, it would be of great benefit for microbiology students. I would recommend this manual for all MBBS students.

I congratulate all the authors and am delighted to encourage and support them in pursuit of their objective. I wish all the authors a grand success.

Dr Anil K Jain
MS FAMS FRCS (Eng.)

Principal
Director-Professor and Head
Department of Orthopaedics
University College of Medical Sciences and GTB Hospital,
Delhi

Foreword

I am indeed honored to write this Foreword for *Microbiology Practical Manual.* I really appreciate the efforts made by my colleagues Dr Shukla Das and Dr Rumpa Saha for understanding the need of our students and in this endeavor enthusiastically preparing this practical manual.

They are our very dedicated teachers with a deep interest in the subject. As examiners, they are well appreciated by the students.

This manual is very well planned and prepared with the objectives to envelop all the psychomotor domains of undergraduate microbiology and to educate the students to accomplish these tasks with ease. It also aims to attain homogeneous learning. Thus it would be of definite benefit to microbiology students. I would recommend this manual to all MBBS students.

I applaud the authors and am pleased to encourage them in quest of their objectives. I wish the authors a grand success.

Dr N P Singh
Director-Professor and Head
Department of Microbiology
University College of Medical Sciences and GTB Hospital
Delhi

Preface

Microbiology Practical Manual provides the MBBS students a comprehensive, reliable and informative approach to all practical aspects of undergraduate microbiology.

This manual contains all images of demonstration slides/specimens and other related items with characteristic features of each, relevant for undergraduate formative training.

For better understanding of the students, we have used some pictures from internet/www.google for which we have acknowledged.

For maintaining uniformity, all practical procedures have been clearly written and objectives are defined to enable students to follow and recall.

We express our sincere thanks to our Principal, Director-Professor Dr A K Jain for his encouragement and for writing the Foreword for this manual. Our heartfelt thanks are also for our Head of Department, Director-Professor Dr N P Singh for his constant support while preparing this manual and contributing for the Foreword. Thanks are also due to M/s CBS Publishers & Distributers Pvt. Ltd., for their cooperation and keen interest in the publication of this manual.

Rumpa Saha
Shukla Das

Contents

Foreword by Dr Anil K Jain .... *v*
Foreword by Dr NP Singh .... *vii*
Preface .... *ix*

Section 1: General Microbiology Practicals

1. Universal Presence of Microbes 3
2. Microscope: General Instructions about Use and Care 5
3. Microscopy and Micrometry 7
4. Methods of Sterilization and Disinfection 11

Section 2: Parasitology Practicals

5. Preparation of Saline and Iodine Wet Mount of Stool Sample 15
6. Formol-Ether Concentration Method for Stool Examination 17
7. Normal Stool Findings 19
8. *Entamoeba histolytica, Entamoeba coli* and *Giardia lamblia* 23
9. Protozoa and Coccidian Parasites 27
10. Preparation of Blood Film 31
11. Morphological Forms of *Leishmania donovani* 37
12. Peripheral Blood Smear Examination for Malarial Parasites 41
13. Eggs of Helminths (Cestodes) 47
14. Eggs of Helminths (Nematodes) 51

Section 3: Bacteriology Practicals

15. Albert Staining 59
16. Ziehl-Neelsen (ZN) Staining 63
17. Antimicrobial Susceptibility Testing 67
18. Description of Growth of Bacteria on Solid or in Liquid Media 69
19. Gram Stain 71
20. *Staphylococcus aureus* 73
21. *Streptococcus pyogenes* 79
22. Gram-negative Cocci 83
23. Culture Media and Biochemical Reactions of Enterobacteriaceae Family ... 85
24. *Escherichia coli* 99

25. *Klebsiella*   101

26. *Proteus*   103

27. *Salmonella*   105

28. *Shigella*   111

29. Non-fermenters: *Pseudomonas*   115

30. Demonstration of *Vibrio, Spirochaete* and *Chlamydia trachomatis*   119

31. Spore Staining and Anaerobic Methods   123

Section 4: Mycology Practical

32. Characteristic Features of Fungi   131

Section 5: Entomology Practical

33. Arthropods of Medical Importance   143

Section 6: Virology Practical

34. Virology Methods   155

Rules and Safety Precautions to be Observed in the Microbiology Laboratory

1. Wash your hands with soap and water after handling the infectious material.
2. Wear laboratory coats in the laboratory.
3. Keep the nails clean and short.
4. Tie up long hair, while working in the laboratory.
5. Avoid eating, drinking and smoking in the laboratory.
6. Decontaminate the working area with appropriate disinfectant after spillage of potentially infected material.
7. Carry-out the laboratory procedure following standard precautions.
8. Avoid mouth pipetting as far as possible.
9. Perform all the laboratory procedures in a way that minimizes the aerosol formation.
10. Bring practical manual in all the practical classes.
11. Draw properly labeled diagrams neatly, get it corrected from your teachers.
12. Leave your microscope and work seat clean before going out of practical lab.
13. Keep your bag away from working tables.
14. Come exactly at 2.00 pm for practical and tutorials.

General Microbiology Practicals

1. Universal Presence of Microbes

2. Microscope: General Instructions about Use and Care

3. Microscopy and Micrometry

4. Methods of Sterilization and Disinfection

Universal Presence of Microbes

Aim: To demonstrate the universal presence of microorganisms on animate and inanimate surface.

Method: Using a sterile swab, swab an area on the table top / on hand between the webs of fingers and inoculate on blood agar culture plate. Leave a plate of blood agar exposed in air for 1 hour, cover and incubate the plates overnight by 37°C. Note the growth of microorganisms on the culture plates the next day.

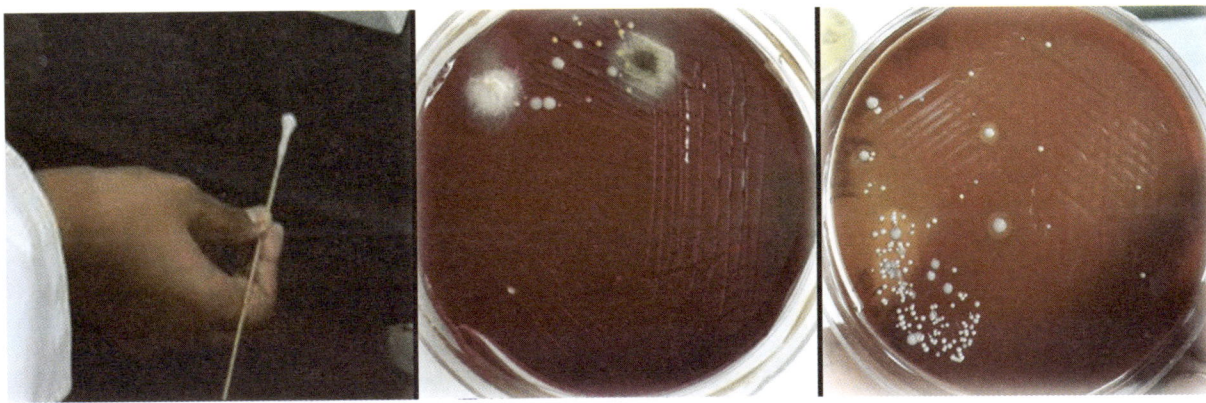

1. On the table top

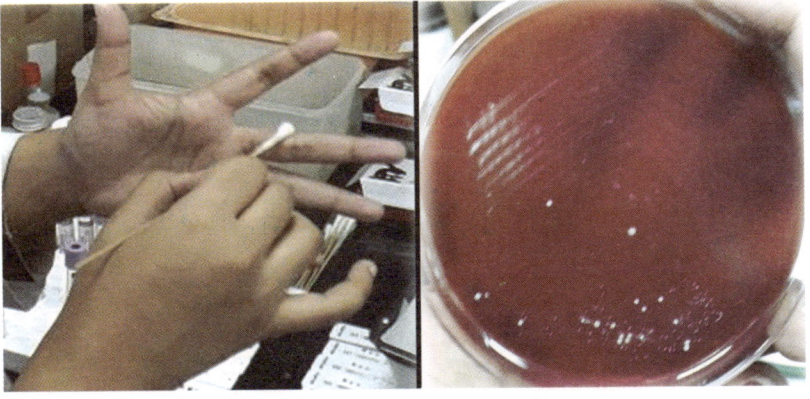

2. Between the webs of fingers

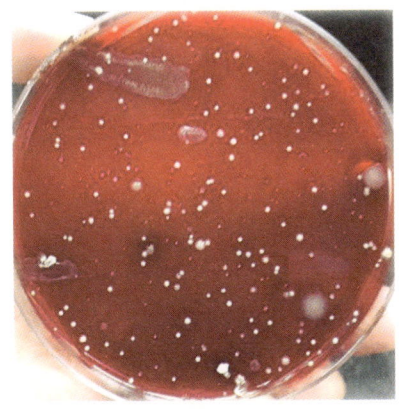

3. From the air after plate is exposed for 1 hour in air

Inference: Microorganisms are present universally.

Signature of Teacher

Microscope: General Instructions about Use and Care

1. Always observe an object with the body of the microscope in a perpendicular position. Do not tilt the microscope.
2. Train yourself to look with both eyes open, to reduce eye strain.
3. Do not attempt to take any part of the microscope apart.
4. Use artificial source of light provided on the work table. Use the plain side of mirror.
5. Never leave oil on the objectives. Wipe gently after the use and if oil has been left on for sometime, wipe with lens-paper or soft cloth moistened with xylene.
6. Do not touch the slide with objective lens. Always focus away from the slide, thus avoiding damage to the lens and slide.
7. Partly close the diaphragm for unstained preparation and keep the condenser down.
8. Always focus first with low power and then swing 'high power' in position and bring object into focus with fine adjustment. These two objectives are used for stool, urine, and hanging drop preparations.
9. Oil immersion lens is used for bacterial preparations, etc. Place a drop of oil on slide, lower the lens to touch the oil and focus with fine adjustment. The condenser should be right up when oil immersion is being used.
10. Objectives are as follows:
    - Lower power   — 16 mm
    - High power   — 4 mm focal length
    - Oil immersion — 1.8 mm

    These figures are working distances or focal lengths and very short in the last two, the fine adjustment must be used for focusing.
11. Magnification

    Usual corrected tube length   = 16 cm = 160 mm

    Distance of image   = 16 cm = 160 mm

    Distance of object   = Focal length of objective

    Using low power and eyepiece (EL) — 10X

    $$\text{Magnification} = \frac{\text{Distance of image}}{\text{Distance of object}} \times \text{Magnification of eyepiece}$$

    $$= \frac{160}{16} \times 10$$

12. Always leave your microscope lenses clean, oil and dust free after you finish your practical.

_____
Signature of Teacher

5

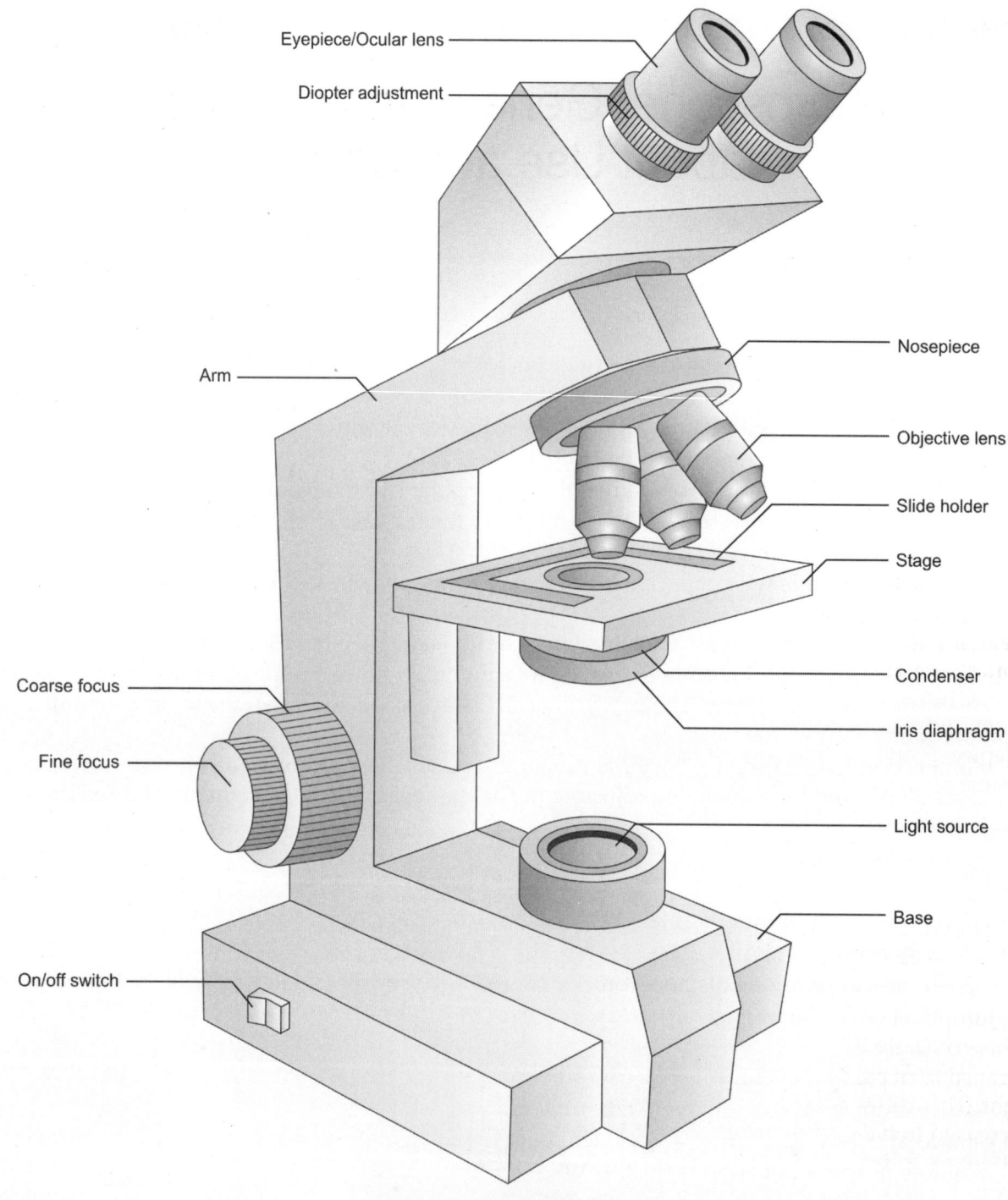

Eyepiece/Ocular lens

Diopter adjustment

Arm

Nosepiece

Objective lens

Slide holder

Stage

Condenser

Iris diaphragm

Coarse focus

Fine focus

Light source

Base

On/off switch

Parts of a Light Microscope

Microscopy and Micrometry

Microscope: Instrument to magnify and resolve microbes and very small objects.

Microscopy: It deals with magnification of object so as to show the finest details of the object.

Principle: The light rays pass through the object, the objective and series of lenses to form a magnified and resolved image of the object. Real, inverted and enlarged image is formed by the objective lens, while virtual erect and enlarged image is formed by eyepiece lens which is seen by the observer.

Parts of a Light Microscope

1. Base—system rests over it.
2. Foot—horseshoe shaped
3. Mirror—directs light in optical system
   Plane mirror to be used for point source of light
   Concave mirror for natural light.
4. Condenser—regulates amount of light entering.
5. Stage—to place the slide.
6. Eyepiece—objects viewed with this.
7. Coarse and fine adjustment screw—for focusing clearly and properly.

Position of Condenser

10X: Lowest
40X: Middle
100X: Highest

Types of Microscope

1. **Light/optical microscope:** Uses visible light and a system of lenses to magnify images of small samples.
2. **Phase contrast microscope:** The phase contrast microscope uses the fact that the light passing through a transparent part of the specimen travels slower and due to this is shifted compared to the uninfluenced light. This difference in phase is not visible to the human eye. However, the change in phase can be increased to half a wavelength by a transparent phase-plate in the microscope and thereby causing a difference in brightness. This makes the transparent object shine out in contrast to its surroundings.
   Uses:
   • Identification of cellular structures.
   • Motility of organisms, cell division can be observed in real time.
3. **Darkfield microscope:** The darkfield microscope creates a contrast between the background and the specimen by adding a special stop condenser. The background appears dark and the specimen bright as the stop condenser prevents all the transmitted light reaching the specimen and only the oblique scattered light reaches the specimen and the lens system.

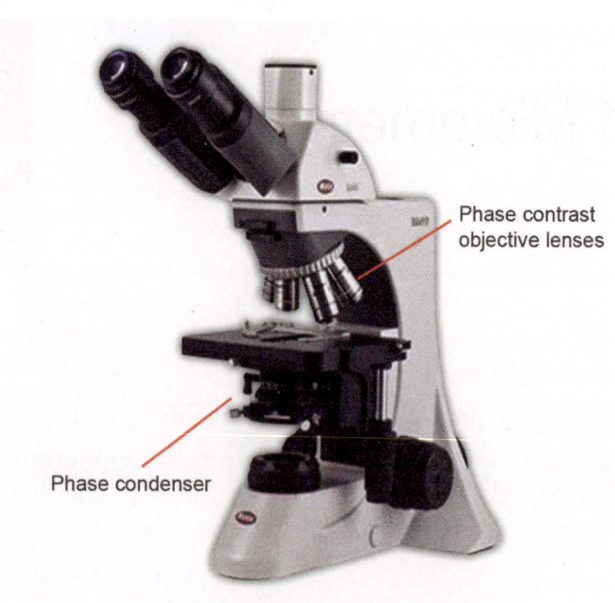

Phase-contrast microscope

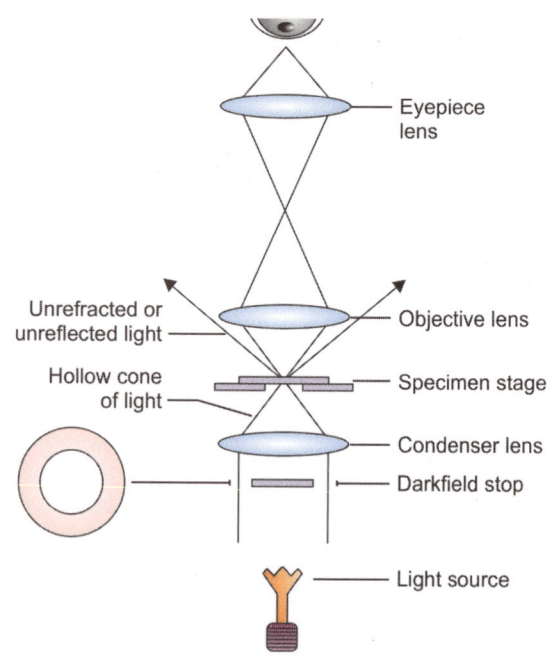

Darkfield microscope

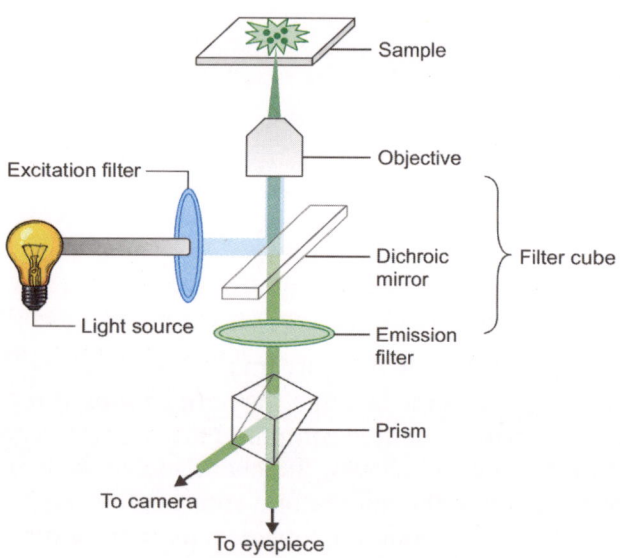

Fluorescent microscope

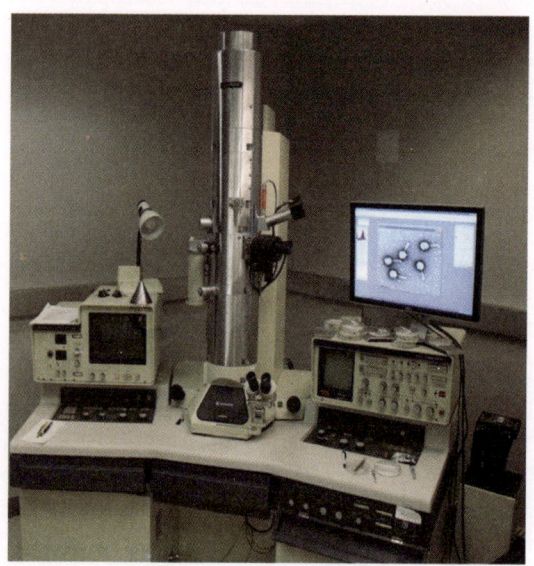

Electron microscope

Uses:
- Identification of Treponemas.
- Motility of organisms.
- Observation of thin fragile organisms which cannot be stained.

4. **Fluorescent microscope:** The sample (cells/organism) is stained with a fluorescent dye and UV light source is used. The UV rays passes through the excitation filter and the objective lens on the sample. The reflected higher wavelength wave passes through the beam splitter and emission filter to reach the eyepiece in a fashion that the wavelength of transmitted ray matches the emission characteristics of the fluorescent dye. So the sample appears colorful on a dark background.
   Uses:
   - Rapid identification of microorganisms, e.g. identification of TB bacilli in sputum, QBC for malaria.
   - Identification of specific protein and DNA in tissue sections.

5. **Electron microscope:** A beam of accelerated electrons is used as a source of light which is passed in a vacuum stack with array of electrostatic and electromagnetic lenses. This beam then passes through the specimen which in part scatters them. This reflected electronic beam carries the structural detail of the specimen and reaches the objective lens which is then further magnified by it. The real image formed is photographically captured and can be seen on a computer screen.
   Uses:
   - High velocity of electrons and low aperture of the EM allow higher magnification up to 0.3–0.5 nm.
   - Visualization of minute cellular detail is possible.
   - Visualization of virus

Micrometry: Measurement of size of microscopic objects is called micrometry.

Basic Principle of Micrometry

Micrometry deals with the measurement of microscopic objects like blood cells, microorganisms, etc.
It has two components: The eyepiece micrometer and the stage micrometer.
1. The eyepiece micrometer is a graduated scale from 0 to 10 without standardized measurement.
2. The stage micrometer is a slide with a microscopic 1 mm scale on it. Each division of stage micrometer measures 1/100th mm, i.e. 10 µm (0.001 mm).

   After focusing both the eyepiece and the stage micrometer, the scales are aligned and total number of stage micrometer division within 100 divisions of eyepiece micrometer are counted. After this, total length of eyepiece micrometer is calculated and divisional measurement is calculated by unitary method. After obtaining the measurement of single eyepiece division the stage micrometer is removed and the slide with the sample is focused. Number of eyepiece division within a single cell is counted and multiplied by the eyepiece division.

   Remarks: The measurement of eyepiece division is not constant and changes with the magnification of the objective and the tube length.

   Example: At 40X magnification, 100 eyepiece divisions are equivalent to 25 stage divisions, i.e.
   100 eyepiece division × size of each eyepiece division (n) = 25 stage divisions × size of each stage division (10 µm),

$$n = \frac{25 \times 10 \text{ µm}}{100}$$
$$n = 2.5 \text{ µm}$$

Focus a Giemsa stained blood slide and calculate number of eyepiece divisions within a RBC.

Suppose, 1 RBC = 3 eyepiece divisions
Then diameter of 1 RBC = 3 × 2.5 µm = 7.5 µm

Signature of Teacher

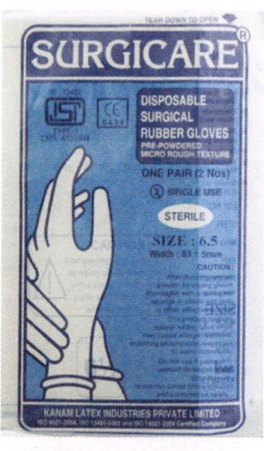

A pair of disposable surgical rubber gloves of size 6.5

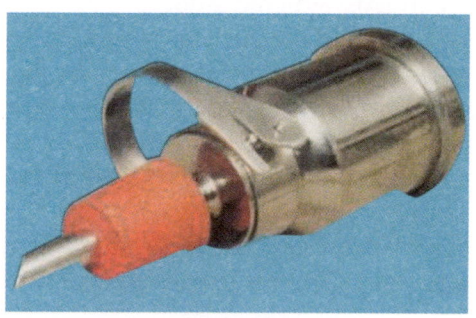

Seitz filter

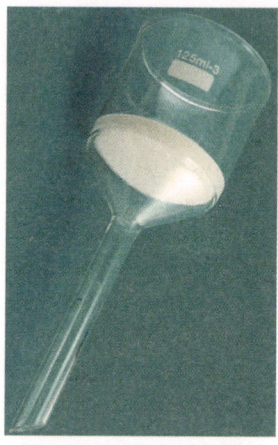

Sintered glass filter

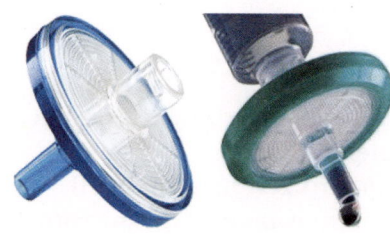

Millipore membrane filter
Available in pore sizes 0.22 µ/0.45 µ

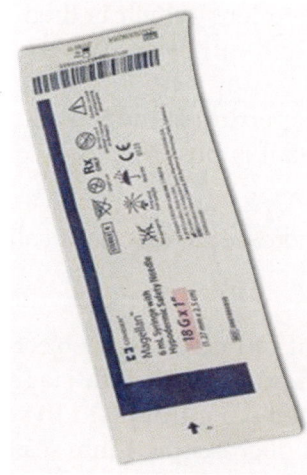

Sterile disposable plastic syringe of 2 ml capacity with 18G hypodermic needle

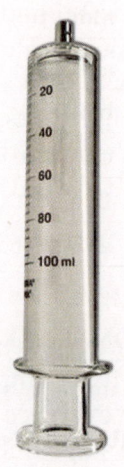

Glass syringe of 100 ml capacity

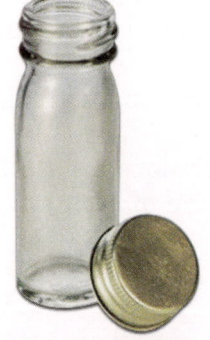

Universal container (McCartney bottle)

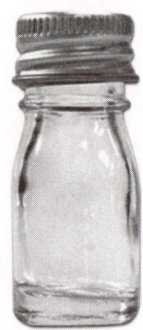

Bijou bottle

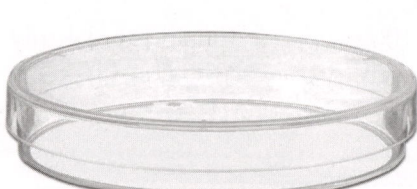

Glass petri plate

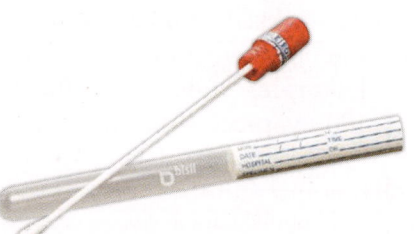

Sterile swab

Methods of Sterilization and Disinfection

METHODS OF STERILIZATION	
METHODS	**EXAMPLE**
PHYSICAL METHODS	
I. HEAT	
1. Moist heat	
a. Below 100°C	Vaccine bath; pasteurization; inspissation
b. At 100°C	Boiling
c. Above 100°C	Autoclave: Dressings, instruments, medias
2. Dry heat	
a. Flaming, red heat	Bacteriological loupe
b. Hot air oven	Lab glasswares, powders, oils, liquid paraffin
II. IONISING RADIATION	
Gamma rays	Disposable syringe needles/gloves/catheters/swabs
III. FILTRATION	
1. Seitz filter	Serum, vaccine
2. Sintered glass filter	Serum, vaccine
3. Millipore filter	Serum, vaccine
CHEMICAL METHODS	
Chemicals: Glutaraldehyde	Endoscopes, Cystocopes
GASEOUS STERILANTS	
Gas ethylene oxide (EtO)	Disposable syringe needles/gloves/catheters/swabs
METHODS OF DISINFECTION	
Alcohols, e.g. 70% ethyl alcohol	In hand-rubs as antiseptics
Phenols, e.g. cresol; lysol	In tuberculosis lab as disinfectant
Halogens, e.g. 1% Na-hypochlorite	Disinfecting blood and body fluids
Aldehydes, e.g. formaldehyde	Preservations of anatomical specimens
Antiseptics, e.g. copper sulphate	As fungicide in lakes and swimming pools

Section
2

Parasitology Practicals

5. Preparation of Saline and Iodine Wet Mount of Stool Sample

6. Formol-Ether Concentration Method for Stool Examination

7. Normal Stool Findings

8. *Entamoeba histolytica, Entamoeba coli* and *Giardia lamblia*

9. Protozoa and Coccidian Parasites

10. Preparation of Blood Film

11. Morphological Forms of *Leishmania donovani*

12. Peripheral Blood Smear Examination for Malarial Parasites

13. Eggs of Helminths (Cestodes)

14. Eggs of Helminths (Nematodes)

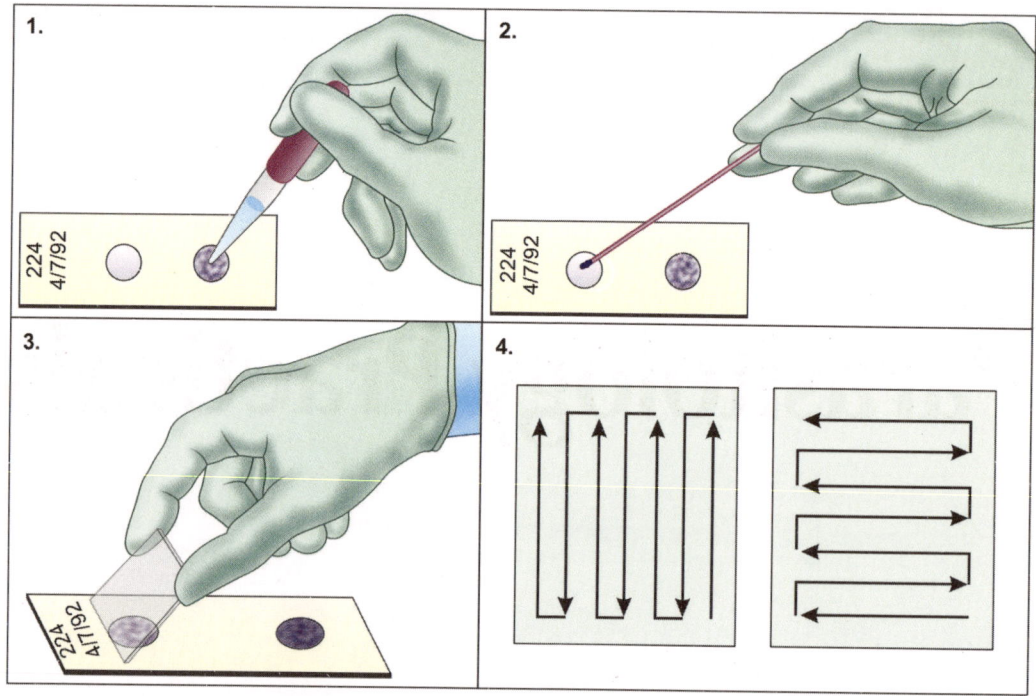

Saline and iodine mount preparation of stool on same slide

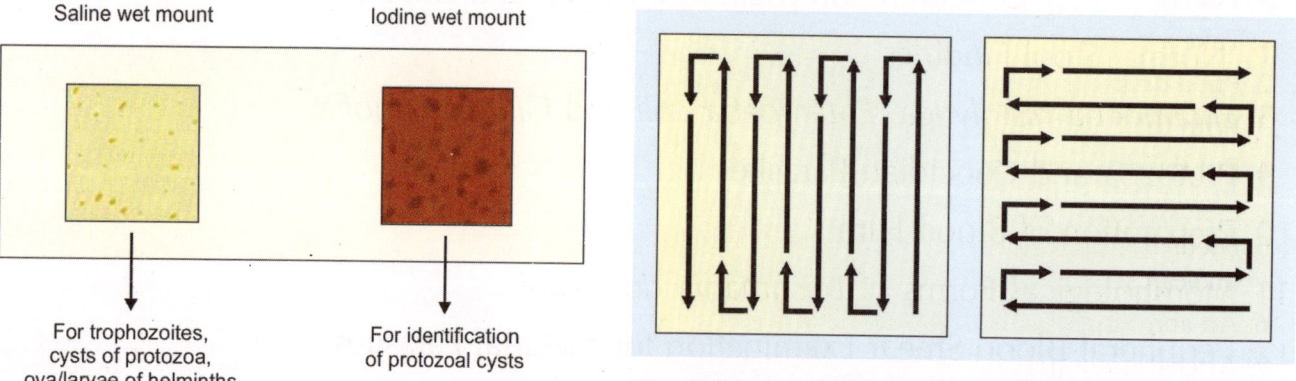

Saline wet mount

Iodine wet mount

For trophozoites,
cysts of protozoa,
ova/larvae of helminths

For identification
of protozoal cysts

Z technique for examination of slide under microscope

Preparation of Saline and Iodine Wet Mount of Stool Sample

Aim: To prepare saline and iodine wet mount of stool sample for diagnosis of ova/cysts.

Materials Required

- Clean glass slide
- Coverslip
- Stool sample
- Clean stick
- Normal saline (NS)
- Lugol's iodine
- Light microscope

Procedure

1. Take a clean slide
2. Put a drop of normal saline on one side of glass slide and of Lugol's iodine on other side.
3. With the help of separate stick, mix the stool sample in both.
4. Put the coverslip over both, drop by making an angle of 45° with slide so that bubble formation is prevented.
5. Focus the slide of normal saline under the low power objective (10X) of a light microscope so that one can see the whole area in low power.
6. An abnormal content or cyst is then focused at high power objective (40X) of a light microscope.
7. After this, iodine slide is focused at low power such that about one-third of slide is focused.
8. Confirm under high power objective.
9. The slides are scanned in a zig-zag (Z) manner.
10. Observe and note your finding first under low power objective (10X) followed by high power objective (40X) of a light microscope.

Note

i. In normal saline, one can appreciate motile trophozoites and bile-stained structures.
ii. In iodine, internal structures especially nucleus is well appreciated but one cannot see motile trophozoites as iodine inhibits motility.

_____
Signature of Teacher

Formol-Ether Concentration Method for Stool Examination

Reagents Required

1. 10% formal saline
2. Diethyl ether
3. Sieve with holes with size of 40 meshes to an inch.
4. Stool for sedimentation

Procedure

- Take stool (~1 gram, i.e. pea sized) in 10 ml distilled water in a conical bottom test tube or centrifuge tube.
- Fix the stopper on the tube and mix thoroughly by shaking for 20 seconds.
- Pass the contents through sieve → centrifuge at 2000 rpm for 1–2 minutes. Decant and discard the supernatant. Final amount of 1.0 to 1.5 ml of sediment should be present.
- Re-suspend the sediment in fresh saline → centrifuge and decant as earlier.
- Add 9.0 ml of 10% formal saline to the sediment and mix thoroughly and add 3.0 ml of ether. Stopper the tube and shake vigorously for 30 seconds.

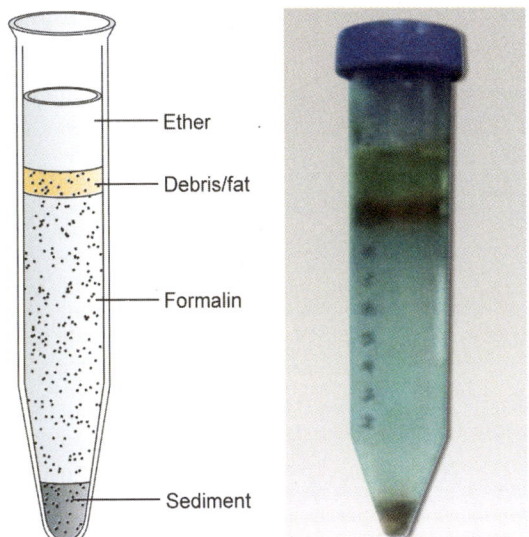

Ether
Debris/fat
Formalin
Sediment

Figures show 4 layers after formol-ether concentration of stool.

- Centrifuge at 3000 rpm for 15 minutes. The liquid column is separated into the following four layers:
  - I. Layer of ether
  - II. Plug of debris
  - III. Layer of formalin
  - IV. Sediment
- Free the plug of debris from the sides of the tube with an application of stick and carefully decant and discard the top three layers. Use a cotton swab to clean debris from the wall of the tube.
- With a pipette, mix the remaining sediment with the small amount of fluid that drains back from the sides of the tube and prepare iodine and unstained mounts for microscopic examination.
- If examination of the specimen is delayed, add 1 or 2 ml of 10% formalin to the sediment and stopper the tube, formalized sediment may be kept for some time if dried. Remove the excess formalin before marking mounts.

_____

Signature of Teacher

Normal stool sample as observed under the microscope

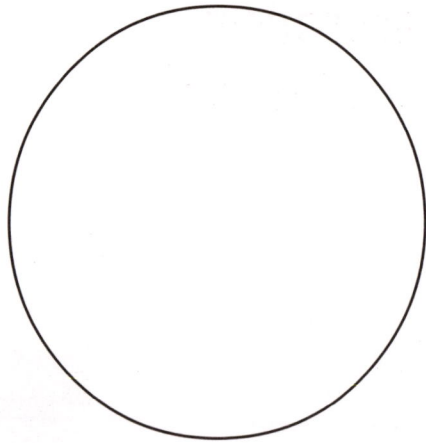

1. Plant hair

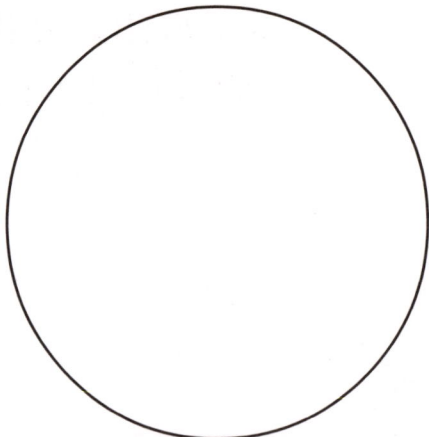

2. Vegetable spiral

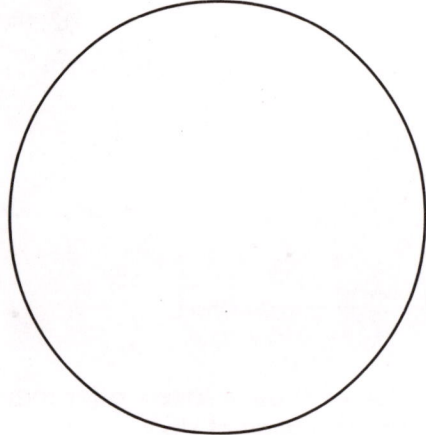

3. Vegetable cell

4. Charcot-Leyden crystal

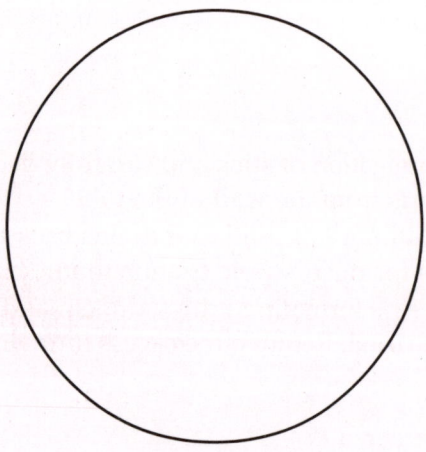

5. Epithelial cells

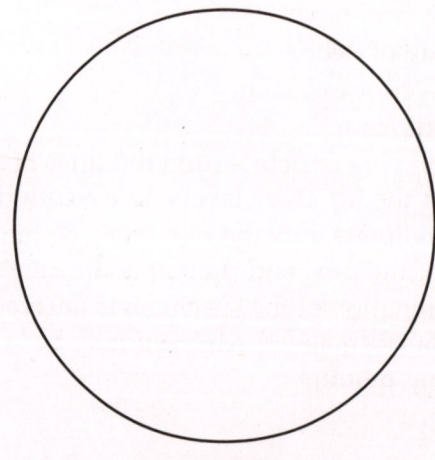

6. Pollen

Normal Stool Findings

The following structures are commonly seen as non-pathogenic findings in a stool preparation.

1. Plant hair
- It has non-descript internal structure
- There is no head or tail region
- May resemble helminth larvae in size and shape (but no diagnostic structures).

2. Vegetable spiral
- They have a ladder like appearance
- Often mistaken with helminth larvae (but they do not have a head or tail region).

3. Vegetable cell
- Round to oval
- Measure up to 150 μm
- Thick cell wall
- Can be confused with helminth egg (interior unorganized).

4. Charcot-Leyden crystal
- These crystals are diamond shaped
- They are eosinophilic breakdown products
- They may be found in sputum also
- Too many in quantity imply some parasitic infection.

5. Epithelial cells
- Single nucleus distinct cell wall
- Resembles amoebic trophozoite

6. Pollen
- Round to symmetrically lobed
- 12–20 micrometer in size
- Thick walled
- Resembling egg of *Taenia* spp. (but smaller with no notable interior structure).

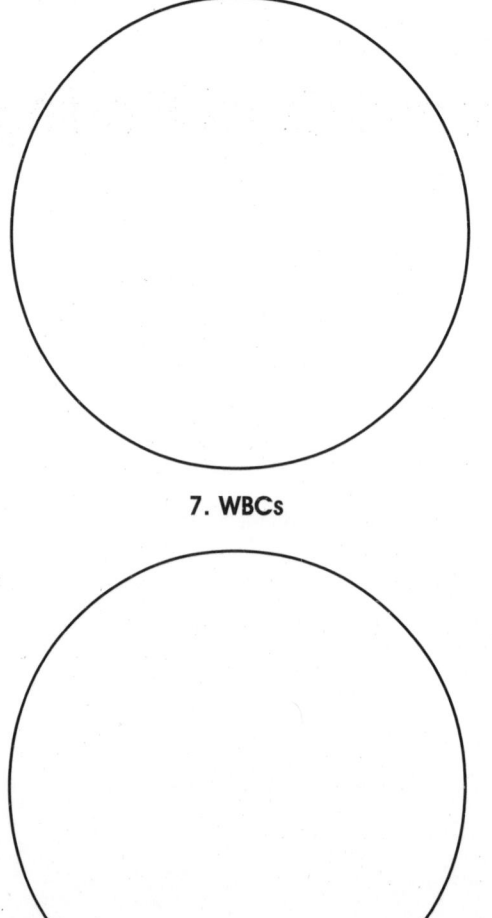

7. WBCs

8. Yeast

7. WBCs

- Size—15 micrometer
- Have 2–4 lobed nucleus connected by chromatin bands
- Can be mistaken with nucleus of *E. histolytica*
- Mononuclear WBC ranges from 28 to 62 μm
- Closely resemble trophozoite of *E. histolytica*
- Degenerated WBCs are pus cells which when present in large numbers imply an invasive diarrhea.

8. Yeast

- Oval structures
- Confused with cysts of *Entamoeba hartmanni, E. nana* but no definite internal structures are seen.

E. coli, *E. histolytica* and *Giardia lamblia* in the given stool sample as seen under microscope

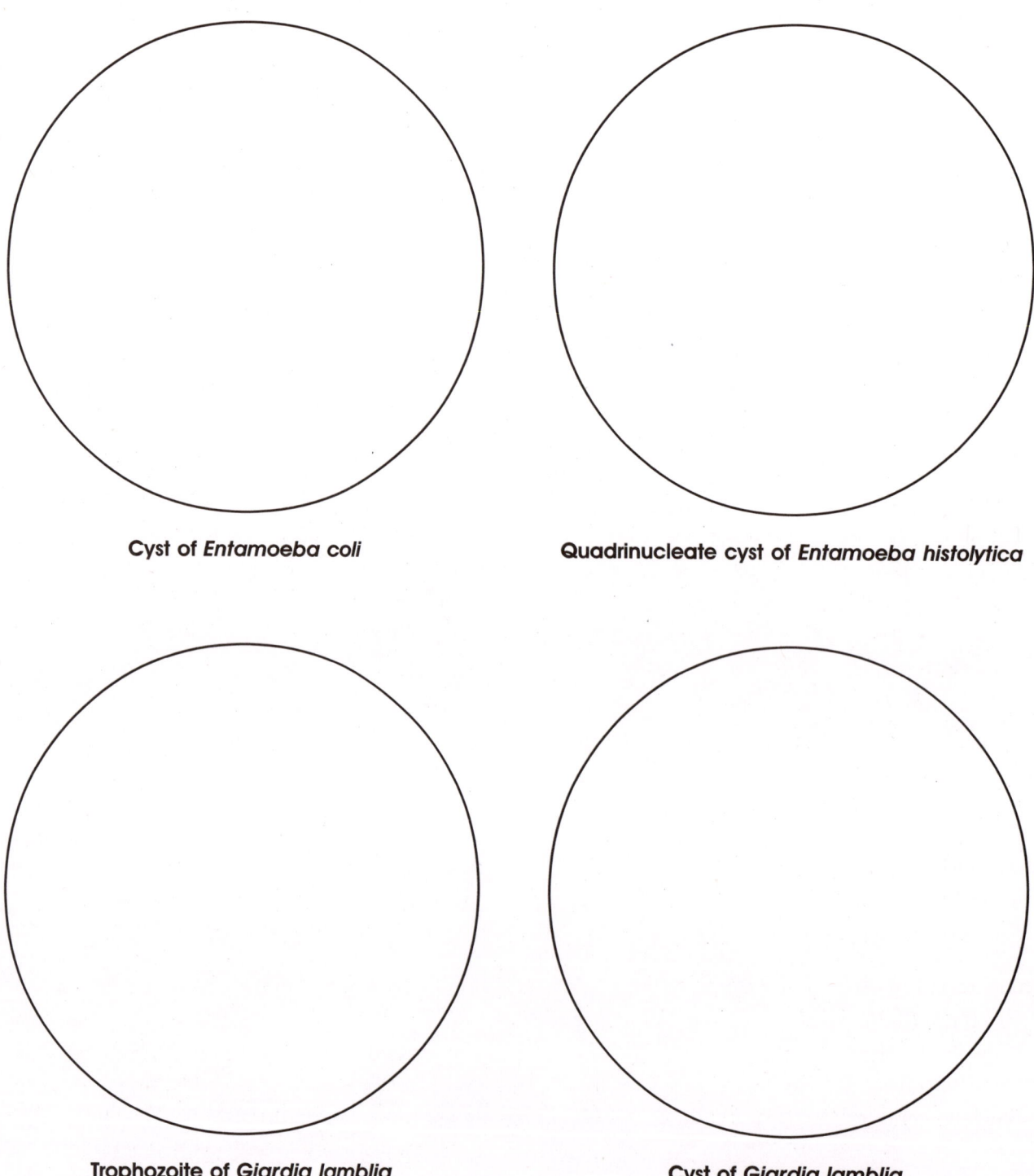

Cyst of *Entamoeba coli*

Quadrinucleate cyst of *Entamoeba histolytica*

Trophozoite of *Giardia lamblia*

Cyst of *Giardia lamblia*

Entamoeba histolytica, Entamoeba coli and *Giardia lamblia*

Aim: To study the characteristic features of the cysts of *Entamoeba histolytica, Entamoeba coli* and *Giardia lamblia* in saline and iodine wet mount preparation of stool.

Prepare a wet saline and iodine mount from the stool sample provided and report your finding.

1. Take a clean slide and put a drop of normal saline on one side of glass slide and of iodine on other side.

2. By the help of separate sticks, mix the stool sample in both.

3. Put coverslip over both drops by making an angle of 45° with slide so that bubble formation is prevented.

4. Focus the slide of normal saline under 10X followed by 40X objective of a light microscope.

5. The slides are scanned in a zig-zag (Z) manner to cover the entire length of coverslip.

6. Observe and note your findings.

Report: Cysts of _____ are seen.

Demonstration

- Giemsa stained slide of cyst of *Acanthamoeba.*
- Formalin preserved specimen of amoebic liver abscess
- NIH media for culture of *Entamoeba histolytica*
- Giemsa stained slide of trophozoites of *Giardia lamblia.*

Characteristic Features of Cyst of *Entamoeba histolytica*

- Round 10–15 μm in diameter; surrounded by highly refractile cyst wall.
- Contains 4 nuclei (quadrinucleate) and central karyosome is present in the nucleus.

Characteristic Features of Trophozoite of *Entamoeba histolytica*

- 10–60 μm in diameter
- Cytoplasm divided into ectoplasm and endoplasm; movement is due to ectoplasmic extension of pseudopodia
- Nucleus spherical, 4–6 μm diameter, karyosome surrounded by clear halo present

Characteristic Features of Formalin Preserved Specimen of Cut Section of Liver Showing (A) Amoebic Liver Abscess

- Caused by *Entamoeba histolytica*
- Usually single and large in size
- Usually located in the postero-superior aspect of right lobe of liver
- Margins are ragged but well defined
- Contains *anchovy sauce* pus
- Amoebae are found in the wall and margins of the abscess cavity

Characteristic Features of Cyst of *Entamoeba coli*

- Round, 15–20 µm in diameter.
- Contains 1–8 nuclei, eccentric karyosome
- Chromatic bodies if present are in the form of slender filaments/pointed threads.

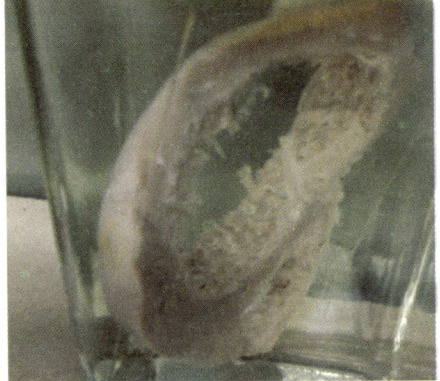

A: Cut section of liver showing ragged wall of a big abscess

Characteristic Features of Cyst of *Acanthamoeba* (B)

- Polygonal/spherical 15–20 µm in diameter
- Double layered cyst wall with central nucleus and large dense karyosome
- Outer wall/ectocyst is wrinkled
- Inner wall/endocyst smooth with pores

Characteristic Features of Cyst of *Giardia lamblia*

- Oval shaped 10–12 µm long and >7–10 µm broad
- Contain 4 nuclei.
- The axostyles diagonally form a division line within the cyst wall.

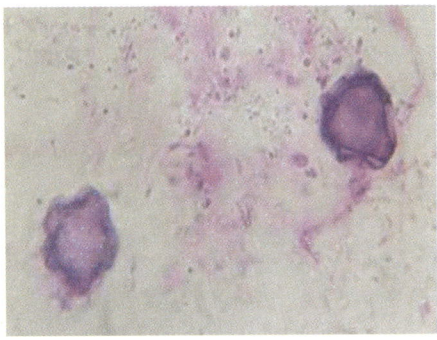

B: Giemsa stained cysts of *Acanthamoeba*

Characteristic Features of Trophozoites of *Giardia lamblia* (C)

- Pear shaped, anteriorly rounded, posteriorly tapering
- 10–12 µm in length, 5–15 µm in width
- Bilaterally symmetrical
- 1 pair of nuclei on each side
- 1 pair of parabasal bodies on axostyles
- 4 pairs of blepheroplasts and flagella.

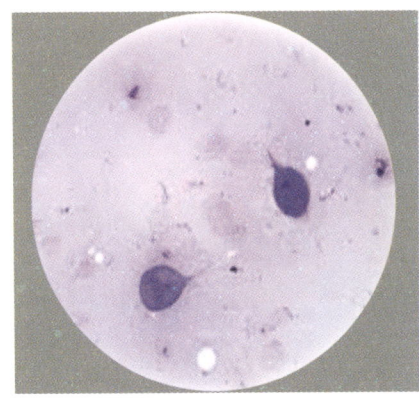

C: Giemsa stained trophozoites of *Giardia lamblia*

Signature of Teacher

Protozoa and Coccidian Parasites

Aim: To study the characteristic features of the coccidian protozoan parasites in stained smears provided.

Demonstration

1. Giemsa stained slide of tachyzoites of *Toxoplasma gondii*
2. Modified acid fast stained slide of oocysts of *Cryptosporidium parvum*
3. Modified acid fast stained slide of oocysts of *Cystoisospora belli*

Characteristic Features of Giemsa Stained Slide of Tachyzoites of *Toxoplasma gondii*

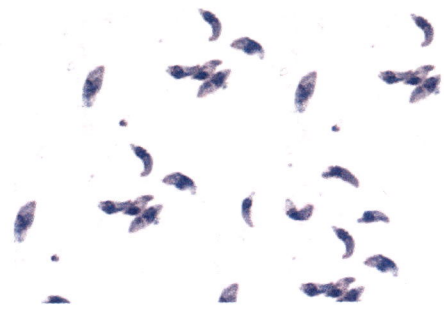

- Crescent shaped with pointed anterior and rounded posterior end
- 6 × 2 μm in size
- Nucleus placed centrally
- Actively multiplying form

Tachyzoites of *Toxoplasma gondii* (Giemsa stained)

Characteristic Features of Modified ZN Stained Slide of Oocysts of *Cryptosporidium parvum*

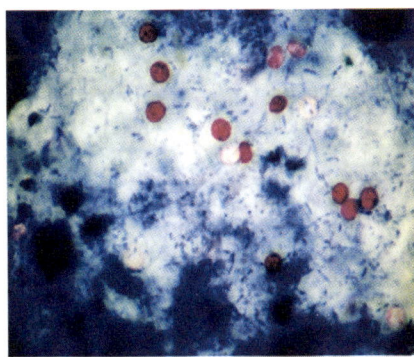

- Characteristically round acid fast structure with variable staining
- 4.5–6 μm in diameter
- Unstained sporulated crescentic forms can be seen within oocysts wall.
- Infective stage in man
- Cause persistent diarrhea in immunocompromised individuals

Oocysts of *Cryptosporidium parvum* (stained by modified ZN technique)

Characteristic Features of Modified ZN Stained Slide of Oocysts of *Cystoisospora belli*

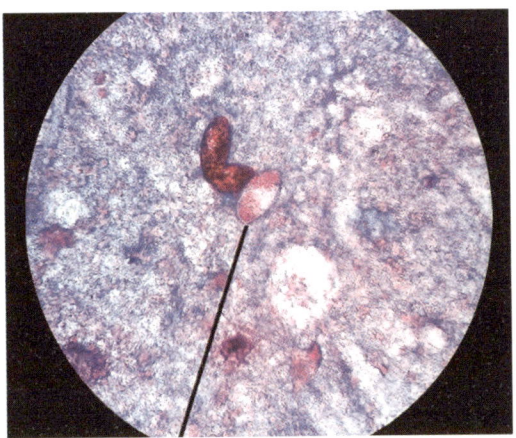

Oocysts of *Cystoisospora belli* (stained by modified ZN technique)

- Characteristically long and oval acid fast structure with variable staining
- Measures 20–33 µm × 10–19 µm
- Mature oocysts have two sporocysts that contain four sporozoites each
- Infective stage in man
- Cause persistent diarrhea in immunocompromised individuals

Signature of Teacher

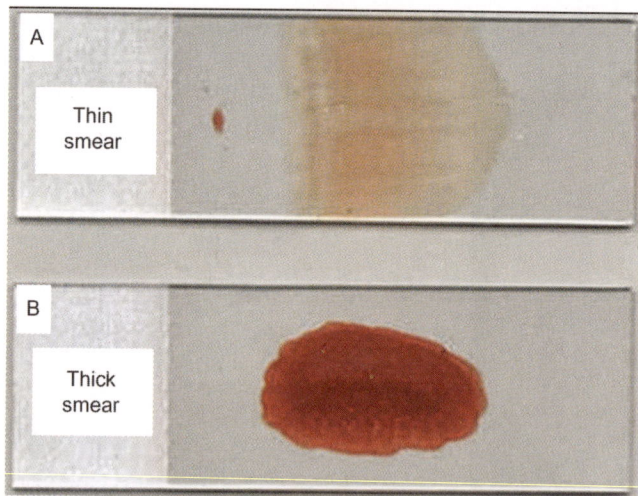

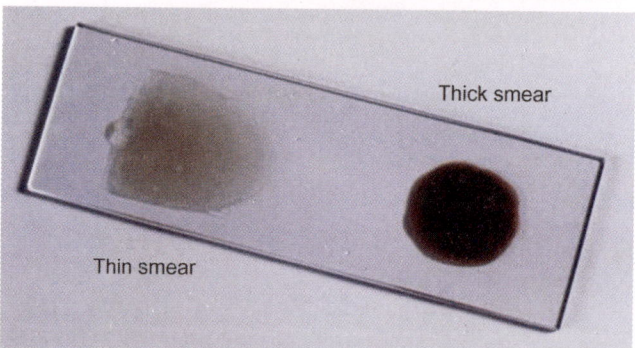

Thin and thick blood smear

Preparation of Blood Film

Aim: To prepare a thick and a thin peripheral blood smear.

THICK FILM

1. Take clean, grease and scratch free glass slides. Clean the second/third finger of the patient's left hand with methylated spirit and completely dry it.
2. Take a sterile needle and puncture the cleaned finger. Squeeze finger gently until a drop of blood exudes.
3. Hold the slide above the blood drop and touch it. Then reverse the slide and spread the blood gently with the corner of another slide to form a circle of half inch. This will form the thick film. Dry it at least for half an hour taking precautions that drying should not be done in sunlight. A moderate thick smear is one which allows one to read print through it.

THIN FILM

1. Take a small drop of blood on a clean grease free glass slide. Hold a spreader at an angle of 45° in contact with the drop of blood. Then push the spreader keeping it at an angle of 30º.
2. Dry the thin film quickly by waving in the air. A properly spread thin film will have a **'tongue'** shape and consists of a single layer of red blood cells.
3. Fix the thin film by dipping in methyl alcohol (pure and acetone free).

DIFFERENT ROMANOWSKY STAINS

I. LEISHMAN'S STAIN

The stain is available commercially in the form of power or tablet. A 0.15% methanolic solution is used for staining.

Staining Method

1. Pour Leishman's stain over the dried film and allow it to remain for 30 seconds.
2. Dilute the stain with twice its volume of neutral or slightly alkaline (pH 7–7.2) distilled water.
3. Allow the diluted stain to remain on the slide for 10–15 minutes.
4. Wash off the stain with running water and examine the dried slide under oil-immersion objective.

II. GIEMSA STAIN

This stain is available as a powder.

Staining Method (Thin Film)

1. Fix the film with methanol or ethanol for 3–5 minutes and allow to dry.
2. Dilute the Giemsa stain by adding 1 ml of the stain to 9 ml of neutral or slightly alkaline (pH 7–7.2) distilled water.
3. Pour the diluted stain over the film and keep for 30–35 minutes.
4. Flush the slide in running tap water and examine the dried slide under oil-immersion objective.

Staining Method (Thick Film)

De-hemoglobinisation to be done before staining is carried out.

1. With **glacial acetic acid and tartaric acid mixture**: The film is flooded with the mixture. As soon as de-hemoglobinisation is complete (indicated by the greyish-white color of the film) the fluid is drained off by tilting. It is then washed thoroughly with neutral or slightly alkaline distilled water so that every trace of acid is removed.
2. In **distilled water** by placing the film in a vertical position in a glass cylinder for 5 to 10 minutes. When the film becomes white, it is taken out and allowed to dry in an upright position.

   Glacial acetic acid and tartaric acid mixture is prepared as follows. 2% glacial acetic acid 4 parts and 2% crystalline tartaric acid 1 part.

III. JSB STAIN

JSB: Staining solution.

JSB I: Methylated blue

Potassium dichromate

Disodium hydrogen phosphate dihydrate

1% sulphuric acid

Distilled water

JSB II: Eosin yellow (water soluble)

Distilled water

Staining Method

1. Fix the thin smear in methanol and dry.
2. Dip the slide in JSB-II for a 1–2 sec.
3. Wash thoroughly to remove excess of eosin
4. Immerse the slide in JSB I for about 45 seconds.
5. Wash in water, dry and examine under oil-immersion objective.

IV. FIELD'S STAIN

Staining solution:

Solution A: Methylene blue
                  Azure I or azure B
                  Disodium hydrogen phosphate (anhydrous)
                  Potassium dihydrogen phosphate (anhydrous)
                  Distilled water

Solution B: Eosin (yellow, water soluble)
                  Disodium hydrogen phosphate (anhydrous)
                  Potassium dihydrogen phosphate (anhydrous)
                  Distilled water

Staining Method

1. The thick film is placed in solution A for 1 to 2 seconds or till the hemoglobin is removed and no trace or green coloring left.
2. It is then removed and immediately rinsed by waving gently in clean water for a few seconds until the stain ceases to flow from the film and glass slide is free from stain.
3. It is then placed in solution B for 1 second.
4. It is removed and rinsed gently in clean water for 2–3 seconds and dried.

Signature of Teacher

Morphological Forms of
Leishmania donovani

Aim: To study the given peripheral blood smear.

1. Giemsa stained slide of peripheral blood smear showing amastigote (LD bodies) form of *Leishmania donovani*
2. Giemsa stained slide of promastigote from a culture of *Leishmania donovani*
3. Mounted specimen of the vector sandfly

Characteristic Features of Amastigote Form (LD Bodies) of *Leishmania donovani*

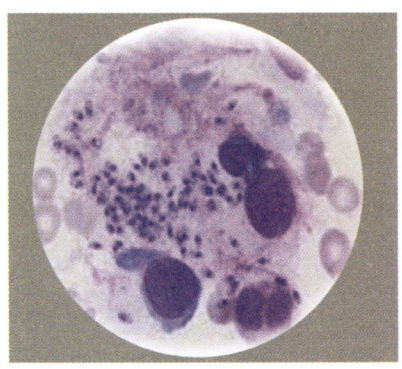

LD bodies

- Oval to round aflagellate form present in RES
- Nucleus is central
- Kinetoplast present
- Axoneme arises from blepheroplast

Characteristic Features of Promastigote Form of *Leishmania donovani*

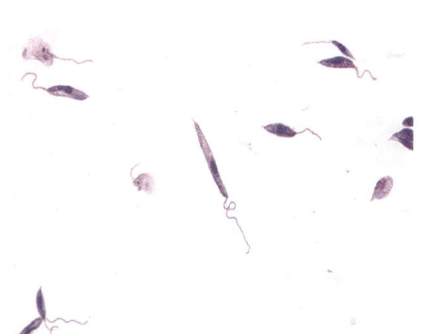

Promastigote form of *Leishmania donovani*

- Elongated, motile extracellular stage
- 15–25 µ × 1.5–3.5 µ
- Nucleus situated centrally
- Kinetoplast lies near the anterior end
- Axoneme arises from blepheroplast which projects from the anterior end of the parasite as free flagellum
- Found in culture media and in insect vector

37

Characteristic Features of Sandfly

- Small insect of 1.5–2 mm in length, body and wings hairy
- Long slender and hairy antennae; palpi and proboscis present
- Thorax bears a pair of wings and 3 pairs of legs
- Wings are upright, lanceolate and hairy, 2nd longitudinal vein branches twice, 1st branching takes place in the middle of the wing
- Sandfly hop but do not fly
- Only females bite, nocturnal biters
- Diseases transmitted—kala-azar, sandfly fever.

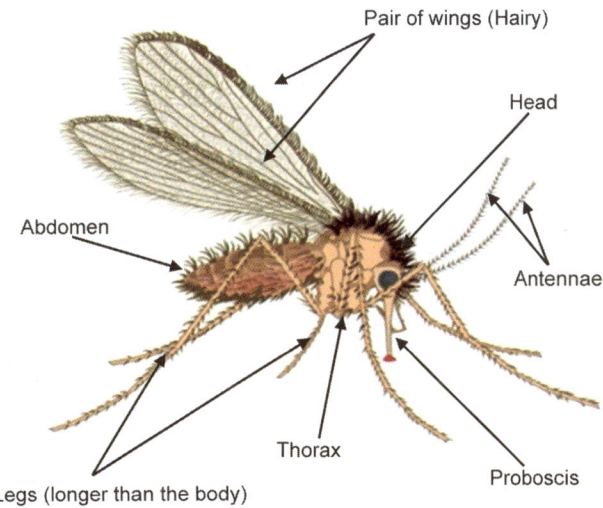

Sandfly

Peripheral Blood Smear Examination for Malarial Parasites

Aim: To study the characteristic features of the different morphological forms of malarial parasites in peripheral blood smear.

- Early trophozite forms/ring stage of *P. falciparum*
- Early trophozite forms/ring stage of *P. vivax*
- Gametocyte of *P. falciparum*
- Gametocyte of *P. vivax*
- Schizont of *P. vivax*

Demonstration

1. Giemsa stained smear of peripheral blood smear showing *Plasmodium falciparum* ring stage, gametocyte.
2. Giemsa stained smear of peripheral blood smear showing *Plasmodium vivax* ring stage, gametocyte, schizont.
3. Specimen of *Anopheles* mosquito.

Characteristic Features of Early Trophozite Forms/Ring Stage of *Plasmodium falciparum*

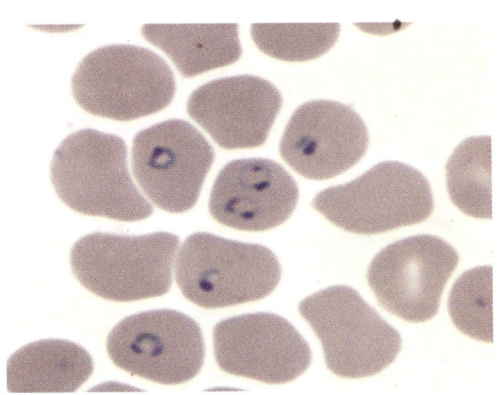

- RBC not enlarged, 1.25–1.5 µm in diameter
- Multiple rings common
- Cytoplasm fine and of regular width throughout the ring
- Parasite may lie along RBC membrane known as accole form.

Early trophozite forms or ring stage of *Plasmodium falciparum*

Characteristic Features of Early Trophozite Forms/Ring Stage of *Plasmodium vivax*

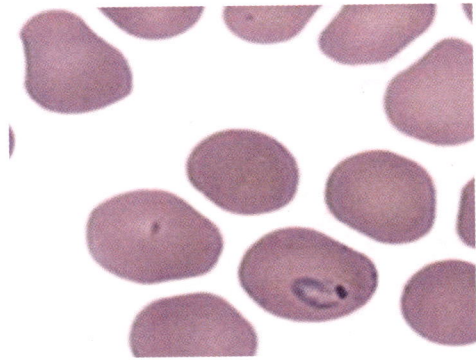

- RBC size enlarged, 2.5 μm in diameter
- Single ring common
- Cytoplasm opposite the chromatin is thicker.

Early trophozite forms or ring stage of
Plasmodium vivax

Characteristic Features of Gametocyte of *Plasmodium falciparum*

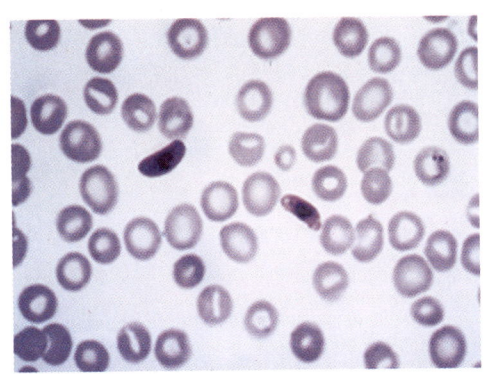

- Crescent shaped (longer and more slender in macro-gametocyte)
- Chromatin diffuse, pigment scattered in large grains (chromatin and pigment more compact in macrogametocyte)
- Pigments aggregate like a wreath round the nucleus
- Cytoplasm stains light blue (dark blue in macrogametocyte)

Gametocyte of *Plasmodium falciparum*

Characteristic Features of Gametocyte of *Plasmodium vivax*

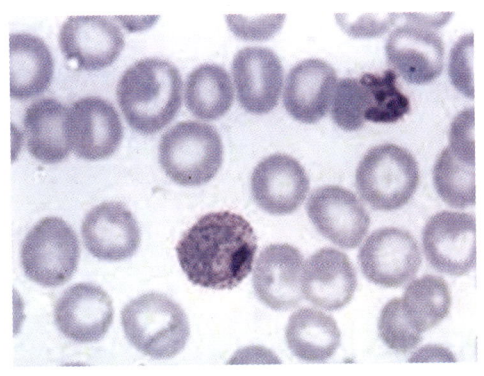

- RBCs spherical, compact, enlarged 1 and ½ to 2 times larger and often distorted
- Diffuse chromatin and coarse brown pigment almost fill the RBCs
- Cytoplasm stains light blue (dark blue in macrogametocyte)

Gametocyte of *Plasmodium vivax*

Characteristic Features of Schizont of *Plasmodium vivax*

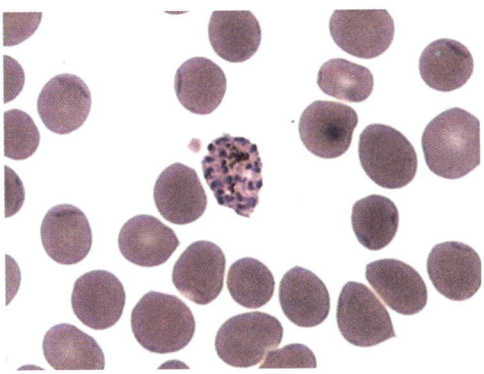

Schizont of *Plasmodium vivax*

- RBC enlarged, size large 9–10 µm in diameter
- Schizont containing merozoites almost fills an enlarged cell

Characteristic features of *Anopheles* mosquito

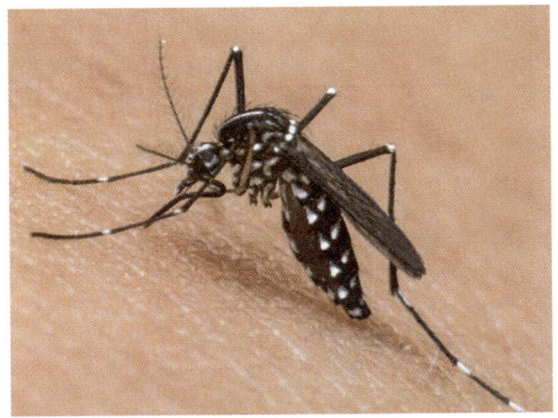

Anopheles mosquito

- When at rest, inclined at an angle to the surface
- Wings spotted (posterior border)
- Palpi long in both sexes
- Breed in fresh water
- Diseases transmitted—malaria, Chittoor virus.
- Important spp. *A. fluviatilis, A. stephensi*

Signature of Teacher

Eggs of *H. nana* and *Taenia* species from stool as seen under microscope

Egg of *Hymenolepsis nana*

Egg of *Taenia* spp.

Eggs of Helminths (Cestodes)

Aim: To study the characteristic features of the eggs of cestodes in saline and iodine wet mount preparation of stool.

Prepare a wet saline and iodine mount from the stool sample provided and report your finding.

1. Take a clean slide and put a drop of normal saline on one side of glass slide and of iodine on other side.
2. By the help of separate sticks, mix the stool sample in both.
3. Put the coverslip over both drops by making an angle of 45° with slide so that bubble formation is prevented.
4. Focus the slide of normal saline under 10X followed by 40X of a light microscope.
5. The slides are scanned in a zig zag (Z) manner to cover the entire length of coverslip.
6. Observe and note your findings.

Report: Eggs of _____ are seen.

Characteristic Features of Egg of *Hymenolepsis nana*
- Spherical/oval, measuring 30–45 µm in diameter
- There are two distinct membranes:

    a. Outer membrane: Thin and colorless.

    b. Inner membrane: Encloses an oncosphere with 3 pairs of hooklets.
- Polar filament emanating from little knobs at either end of embryophore
- Floats on saturated solution of common salt.

Characteristic Features of Egg of *Taenia* **spp.**
- Spherical and brown colored as bile stained
- 31 to 43 µm diameter.
- Embryophore is brown, thick walled and radially striated.
- Contains a hexacanth embryo (oncosphere) with 3 pairs of hooklets.
- Does not float in saturated solution of common salt.

Demonstration

1. Specimen of an adult tapeworm
2. Scolex of *Taenia* mounted on slide
3. Gravid proglottid of *Taenia* mounted on slide
4. Specimen of *Fasciola hepatica*

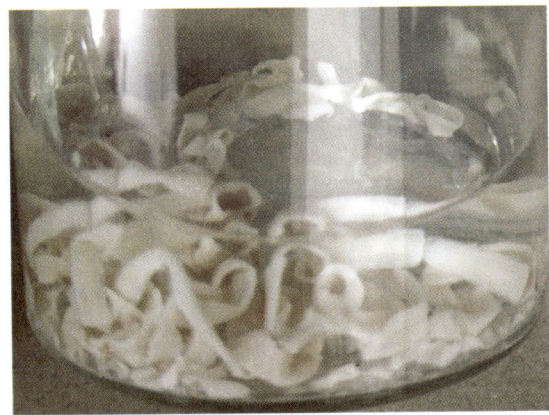

1. Specimen of tapeworm

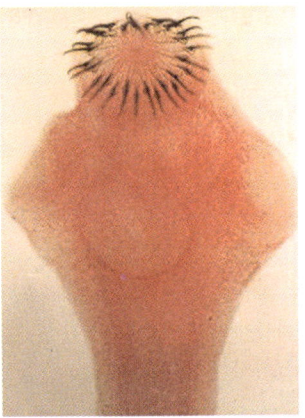

2. Characteristic features of scolex of *Taenia*: Globular in shape with 4 suckers and rounded rostellum armed with double rows of 22 to 36 large and small hooks.

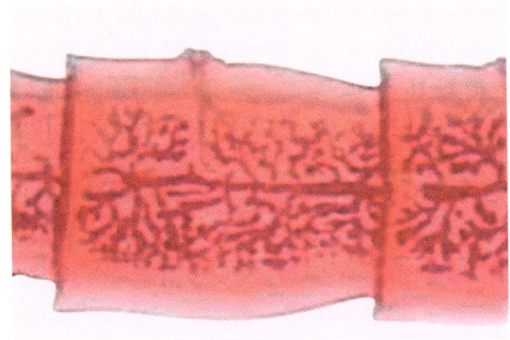

3. Gravid proglottid of *Taenia solium*

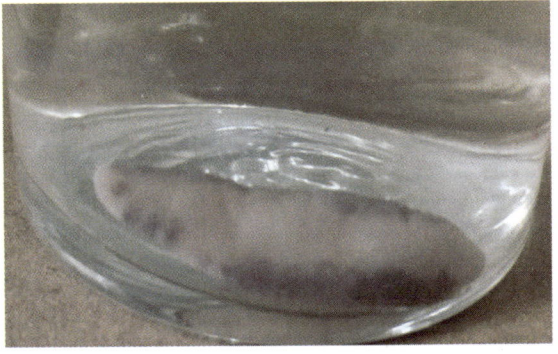

4. Specimen of *Fasciola hepatica*

Signature of Teacher

Eggs of nematodes from stool as seen under microscope

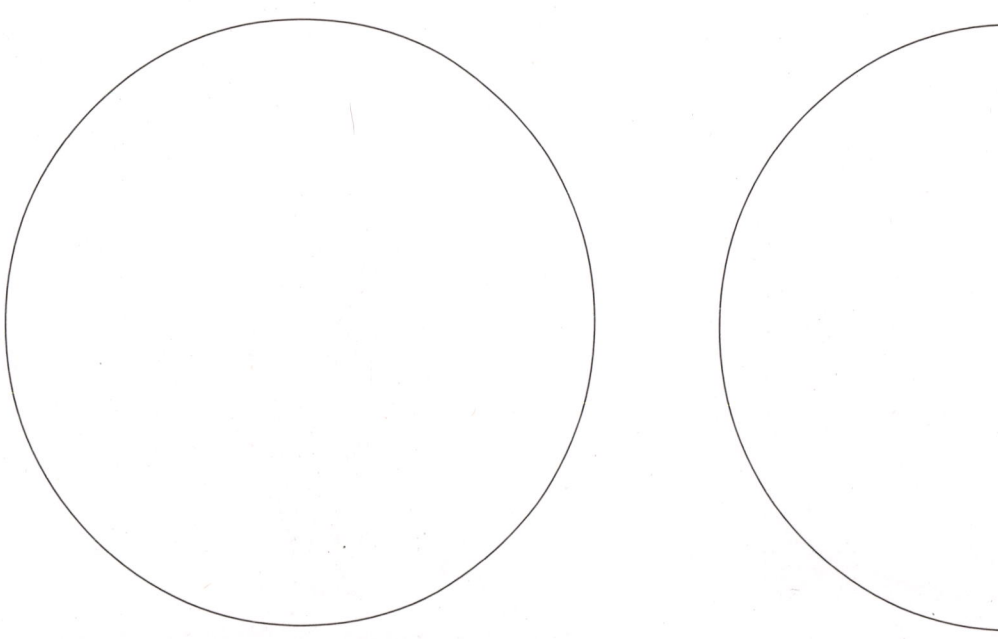

Fertilized egg of *Ascaris lumbricoides*

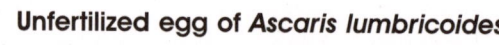

Unfertilized egg of *Ascaris lumbricoides*

Egg of *Ancylostoma duodenale*

Egg of *Trichuris trichiura*

Eggs of Helminths (Nematodes)

Aim: To study the characteristic features of the eggs of intestinal nematodes (*Ascaris lumbricoides, Ancylostoma duodenale and Trichuris trichiura*) in saline and iodine wet mount preparation of stool.

Prepare a wet saline and iodine mount from the stool sample provided and report your finding.

1. Take a clean slide and put a drop of normal saline on one side of glass slide and of iodine on other side.
2. By the help of separate sticks, mix the stool sample in both.
3. Put the coverslip over both drops by making an angle of 45° with slide so that bubble formation is prevented.
4. Focus the slide of normal saline under 10X followed by 40X of a light microscope.
5. The slides are scanned in a zig-zag (Z) manner to cover the entire length of coverslip.
6. Observe and note your findings.

Report: Eggs/ova are seen. Report whether bile stained or non-bile stained.

Characteristic Features of Egg of *Trichuris trichiura*

- Size 50 µm in length and 25 µm in breadth.
- Color is brown, has a double shell. The outer one is bile stained.
- Barrel shaped with a mucous plug at each hole.
- Contain an unsegmented ovum.

Characteristic Features of Egg of *Ascaris lumbricoides*

- Round/oval in shape 60–75 µm in length by 40–55 µm in breadth.
- Bile stained and brown in color.
- Surrounded by thick transparent shell.
- Contain large conspicuous unsegmented ovum with eresentic space at each pole (fertilized egg). In unfertilized egg ovum is atrophied.

Characteristic Features of Egg of *Ancylostoma duodenale*

- Eggs are oval/elliptical measuring 60 µm in length and 40 µm in width.
- Not bile stained surrounded by thin transparent hyaline shell.
- They possess a segmented ovum with usually four blastomeres.
- There is a clear space below ovum segment and the eggshell.
- Egg floats in saturated salt solution.

Demonstration

1. Mounted slide of egg of *Enterobius vermicularis* (thread/pinworm)
2. Mounted slide of adult *Trichuris trichiura* (whip worm)
3. Specimen of *Dracunculus medinensis* (guinea worm)
4. Specimen of *Ascaris lumbricoides* (round worm)
5. NIH swab
6. Giemsa stained slide of peripheral blood smear showing microfilaria.

Characteristic Features of Egg of *Enterobius vermicularis*

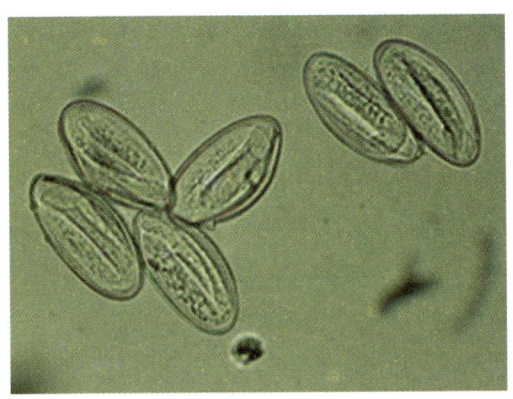

Eggs of *Enterobius vermicularis*

- Non-bile stained
- Asymmetrical in shape being plano-convex, i.e. flattened on one side and convex on outer side.
- Measures about 50–60 μm × 30 μm.
- Surrounded by transparent shell contains a coated tadpole like larva.

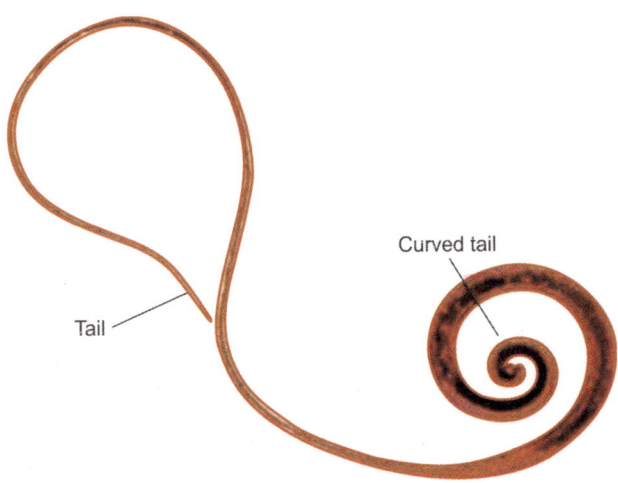
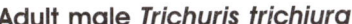

Curved tail

Tail

Adult male *Trichuris trichiura*

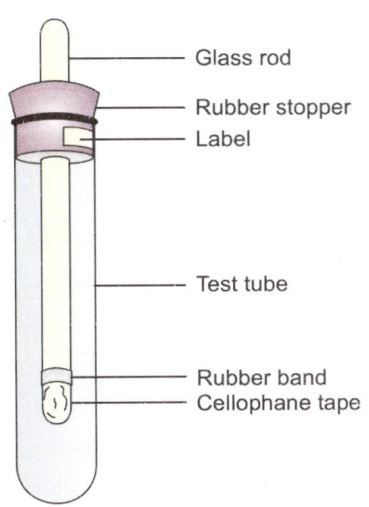

Glass rod

Rubber stopper

Label

Test tube

Rubber band

Cellophane tape

NIH swab

Characteristic Features of Microfilaria (Tissue nematode in Giemsa stained slide of peripheral blood)
- It has a blunted head and pointed tail which is much longer and covered by a hyaline sheath. Nuclei appear as granules in the central axis.
- The tail tip is free from nuclei.
- Periodicity-nocturnal
- Causes lymphatic filariasis transmitted by *Culex* mosquitoes.

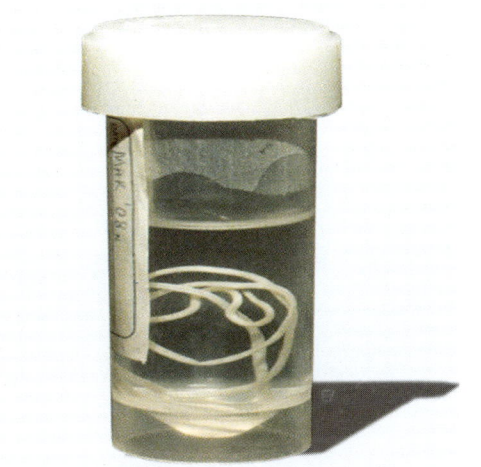

Specimen of guineaworm

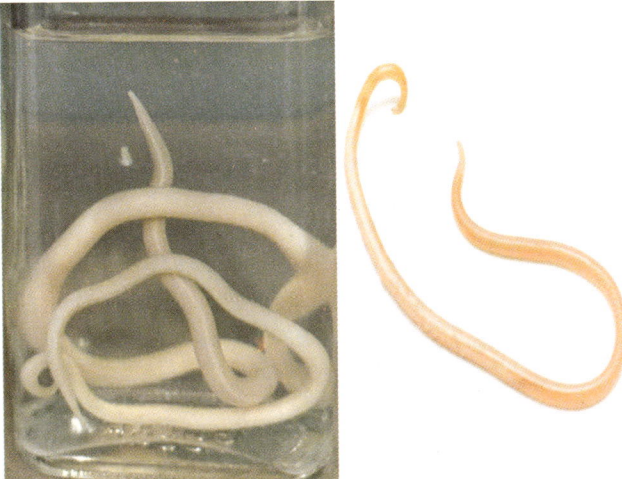

Specimen of roundworm

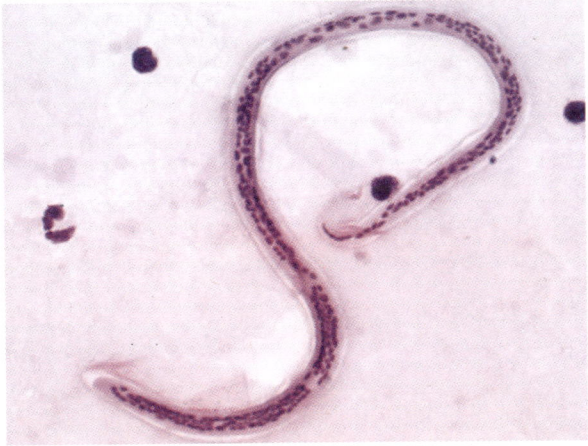

Peripheral blood smear showing microfilaria

Signature of Teacher

Section

3

Bacteriology Practicals

15. Albert Staining

16. Ziehl-Neelsen (ZN) Staining

17. Antimicrobial Susceptibility Testing

18. Description of Growth of Bacteria on Solid or in Liquid Media

19. Gram Stain

20. *Staphylococcus aureus*

21. *Streptococcus pyogenes*

22. Gram-negative Cocci

23. Culture Media and Biochemical Reactions of Enterobacteriaceae Family

24. *Escherichia coli*

25. *Klebsiella*

26. *Proteus*

27. *Salmonella*

28. *Shigella*

29. Non-fermenters: *Pseudomonas*

30. Demonstration of *Vibrio, Spirochaete and Chlamydia trachomatis*

31. Spore Staining and Anaerobic Methods

Morphology of *Corynebacterium diphtheriae* seen under microscope

Appearance of *Corynebacterium diphtheriae* on Albert staining

Albert Staining

Aim: To study the characteristic features of *Corynebacterium diphtheriae* on Albert staining from throat swab of a suspected case diphtheria.

Constituents of Albert Stain

Albert A

- Toludine blue
- Malachite green
- Glacial acetic acid
- Alcohol (95% ethanol)
- Distilled water

Albert B

- Iodine
- Potassium iodide (KI)
- Distilled water

Procedure of Albert Staining

1. Heat fix the provided slide.
2. Cover the slide with Albert A (through filter paper) for 5 min.
3. Drain the slide. Do not wash.

   Cover the slide with Albert B for 4 min.
4. Drain the slide and wash gently with tap water and then dry.
5. Observe under 100X oil immersion objective.

Observation

Green colored bacilli seen with bluish black metachromatic granules at the poles.
The bacilli are arranged in Chinese letter or cuneiform pattern, i.e. V or L shaped.

Report

Microorganisms morphologically resembling *Corynebacterium diphtheriae* are seen.

Demonstration of Culture Media for *C. diphtheriae*

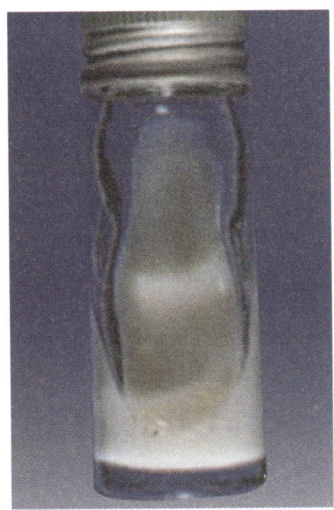

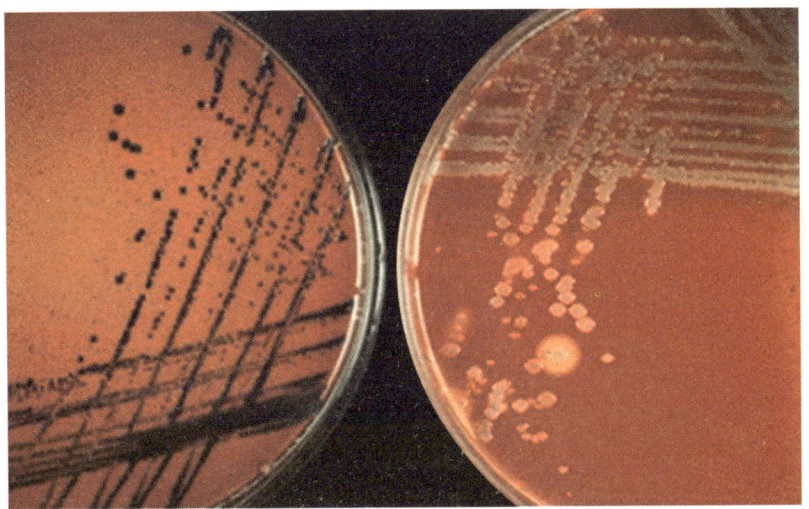

Loeffler's serum slope (LSS):
Contains 70% bovine serum.
Smear prepared from water of condensation.

Corynebacterium diphtheriae forms black colonies on tellurite agar (left), on blood agar colonies appear white (right). Potassium tellurite blood agar (blood agar with 0.04% potassium tellurite).

Acid fast bacilli in ZN stained sputum smear

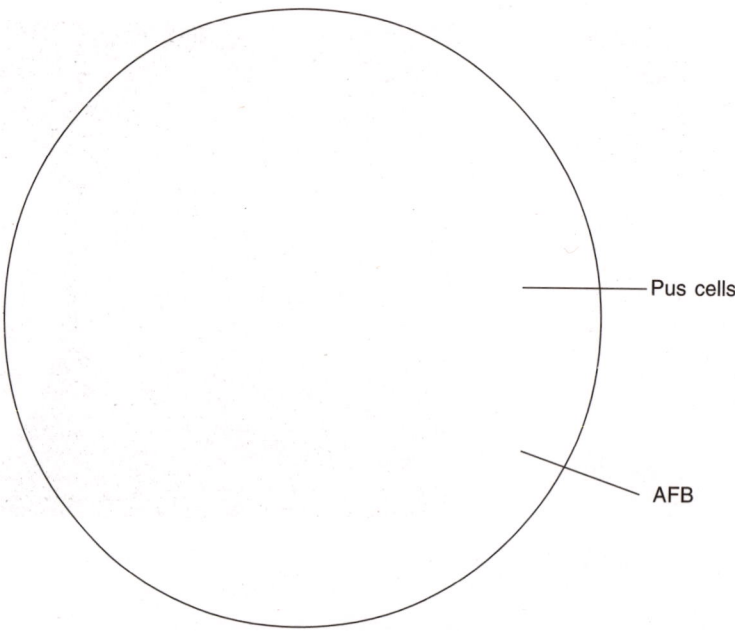
— Pus cells

— AFB

Appearance of acid fast bacilli on ZN staining

Ziehl-Neelsen (ZN) Staining

Aim: To study the morphological features of *Mycobacterium tuberculosis* on ZN staining of a sputum smear and report the findings.

Constituents of Ziehl-Neelsen (ZN) Stain

- **Primary stain** — carbol fuchsin 0.3% (basic fuschin + phenol + 95% alcohol)
- **Decolorizer** — 20% H_2SO_4
- **Counter stain** — 2% methylene blue

Procedure

1. Heat fix the provided slide and keep on slide rack.
2. Flood slide with carbol fuchsin 0.3% and heat the undersurface of the slide with bunsen burner flame only till fumes appear then remove heat. Continue this procedure for 8 min.
3. Drain off the stain from the slide. Do not wash.
4. Decolorize with 20% H_2SO_4 till the pink stain fades.
5. Drain the slide and wash gently with tap water.
6. Counterstain with 2% methylene blue.
7. Wash gently with tap water and dry.
8. Observe under 100X oil-immersion objective.

Observation

Reddish-pink colored bacilli with beaded appearance seen against a blue background showing numerous pus cells.

Report

Smear is positive for acid fast bacilli (AFB).

Demonstration

- To study morphological features of *Mycobacterium leprae* from the stainded slit skin smear provided.
- To study growth characteristics of *Mycobacterium tuberculosis* and atypical mycobacteria on Lowenstein Jensen (LJ) media.

Mycobacterium leprae is uncultivable in artificial culture media but can only be maintained in the following animals.

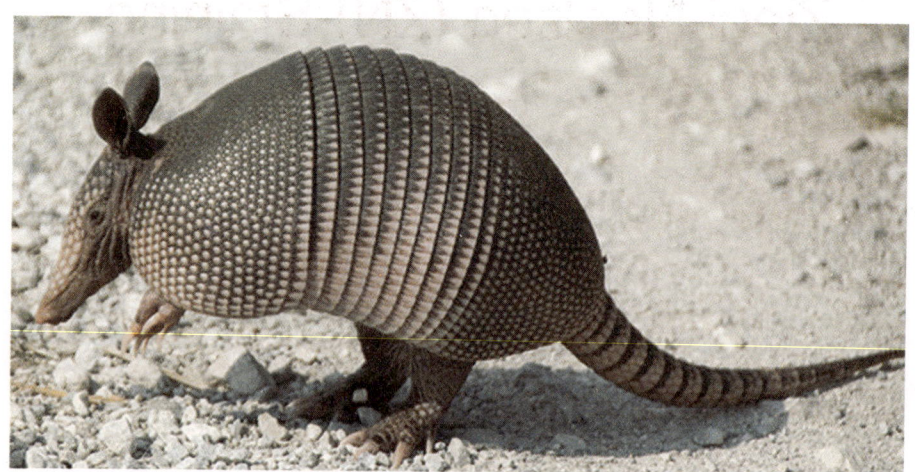

9-banded Armadillo

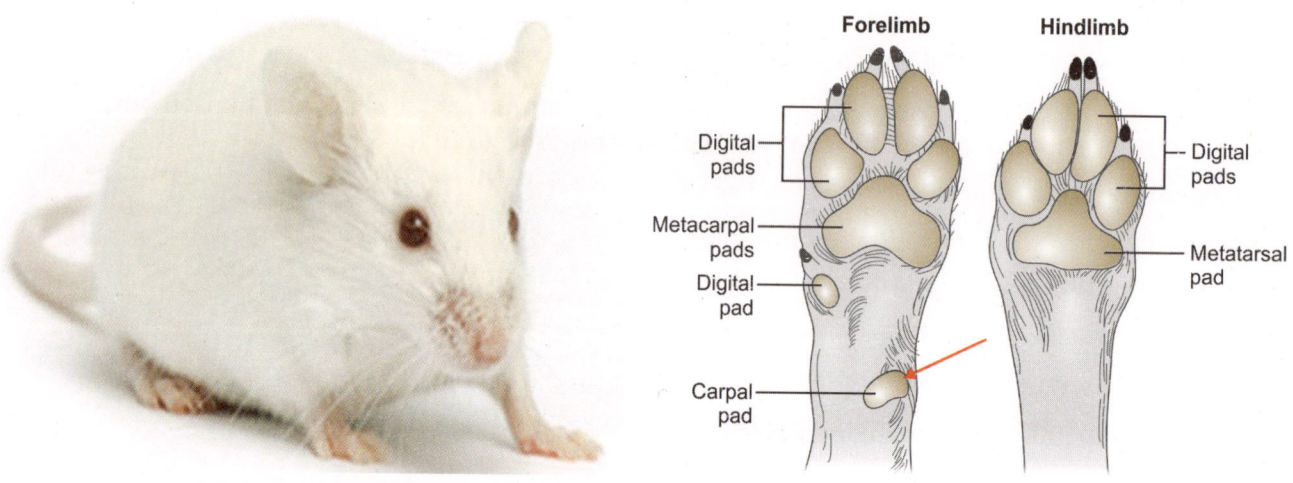

Mouse footpad

Morphological Features of *Mycobacterium leprae* from Stained Slide of a Slit Skin Smear Using 5% H$_2$SO$_4$ as Decolorizer

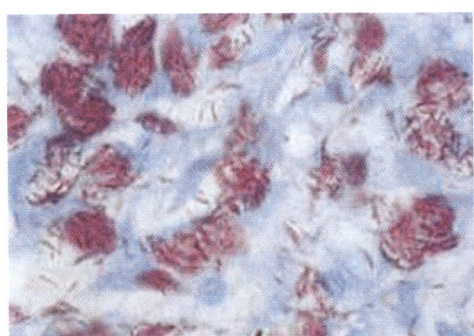

- Red colored bacilli with beaded appearance seen in globi or clumps

ZN stained slide of *Mycobacterium leprae*

Growth Characteristics of *Mycobacterium tuberculosis* and Atypical Mycobacteria on LJ (Lowenstein Jensen) Medium

- *Mycobacterium tuberculosis* growth appears as rough, tough and buff colored colonies against the green background of the LJ media.
- Atypical mycobacteria on LJ medium grows as yellow pigmented colonies against the green background of the LJ media.
- Sensitivity testing for *M. tuberculosis* is also done on LJ media.

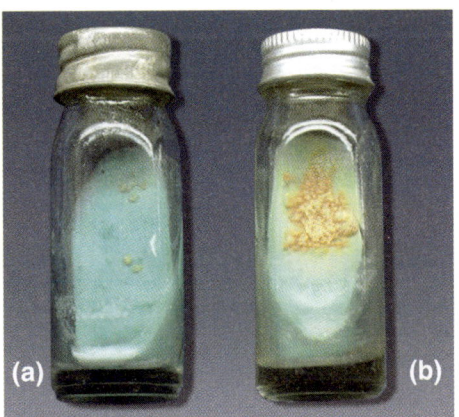

Growth characteristics of (a) *M. tuberculosis* and (b) Atypical mycobacteria

LJ Media: Constituents and Function

- Malachite green (acts as a selective agent; green color permits easy identification of buff colonies)
- Egg (solidifying agent; provides fatty acids and proteins for metabolism of mycobacteria)
- Glycerol (carbon source and favorable to the growth of human type tubercle bacillus while being unfavorable to the bovine type)
- L-asparagine (nitrogen and vitamin source)
- Mono patassium phosphate and magnesium sulphate enhance growth of organism and act as buffers.

Signature of Teacher

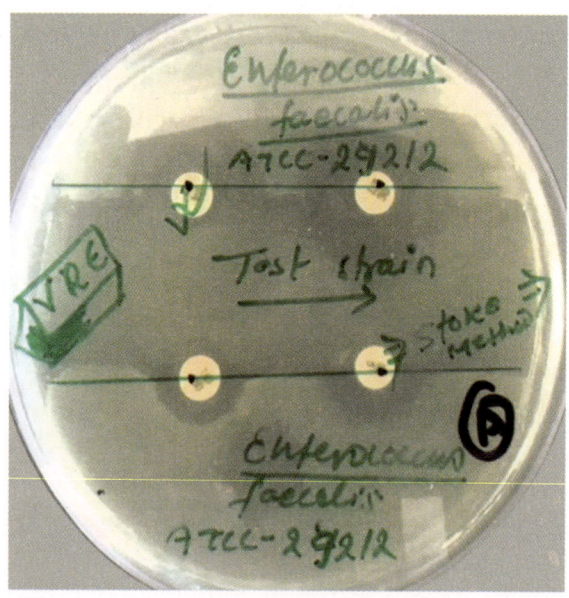

Stokes method: Test strain in centre and control strains above and below

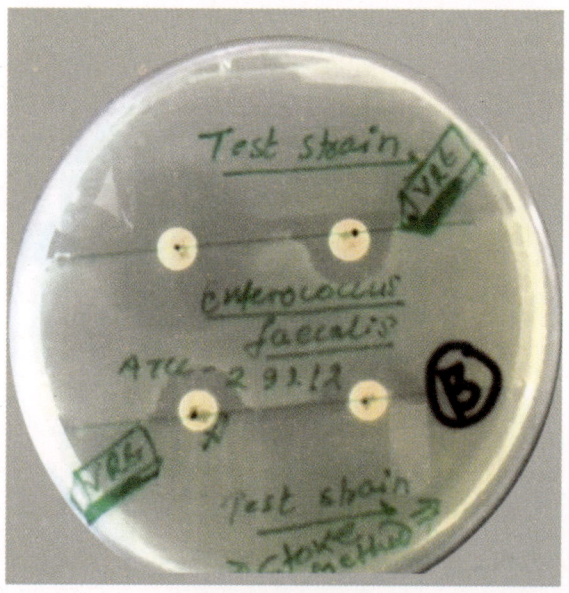

Modified Stokes method: Control strains in centre and test strains above and below. Two separate strains can be tested.

Antimicrobial Susceptibility Testing

Aim: Antimicrobial susceptibility testing (AST) measures the ability of an antimicrobial agent to inhibit growth of microorganism *in vitro*. It is an essential step for properly treating infectious diseases and monitoring antimicrobial resistance (AMR) in various pathogens.

Minimum inhibitory concentration (MIC) is the lowest concentration of an antimicrobial that will inhibit the visible growth of a microorganism following overnight incubation.

Diffusion Method

- Media used: **Müeller Hinton agar**
- Methods used:
  - **Kirby-Bauer method** (using controls ATCC *S. aureus* 25923, *E. coli* 25922, *Pseudomonas* 27853)
  - **Stokes method** (controls NCTC *S. aureus* 6571, *E. coli* 10418, *Pseudomonas* 10662)
  - **E-test** using E-strip

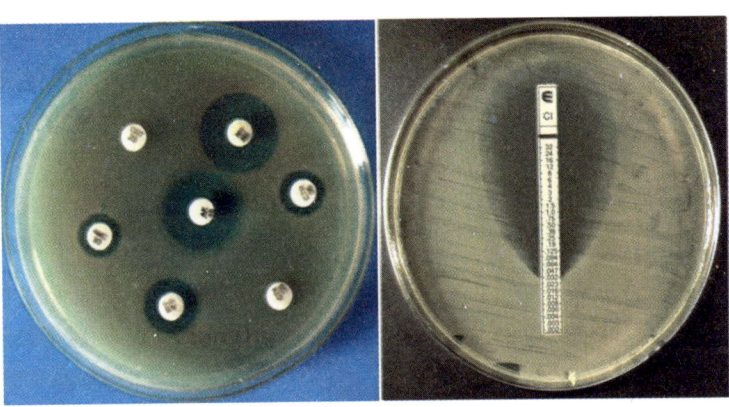

Kirby-Bauer method   **E-test**

Dilution Method

- Agar dilution
- Broth dilution: Macro broth dilution and micro broth dilution

Automated Systems Used

- Microscan walkaway
- Vitek 1 and 2.
- Sensititre

_____
Signature of Teacher

Description of Growth of Bacteria on Solid or in Liquid Media

Aim: To describe colony characteristics of bacterial growth on solid and lequid media.

Description of Colonies on Solid Media

1. Name of the media	:	Blood agar, MacConkey agar, etc.
2. Shape	:	Circular, irregular, radial.
3. Size	:	In millimeters (approx.), pinpoint, pinhead
4. Elevation	:	Raised, low convex, dome shaped, umbonate
5. Surface	:	Smooth, rough, granular, dull or glistening
6. Edge	:	Entire, crenate, spreading
7. Color	:	Colored by reflected and transmitted light, fluorescent
8. Opacity	:	Transparent, translucent or opaque
9. Consistency	:	Butyrous/mucoid/friable
10. Emulsifiability	:	Easy or difficult
11. Pigment	:	Pigmented—diffusible or non-diffusable/non-pigmented
12. Change in medium	:	Haemolysis on blood agar
13. Odour	:	Present seminal/fishy/earthy or absent

Growth in Liquid Medium

1. Degree	:	None/Scanty/Moderate/Abundant
2. Turbidity	:	Present or absent
3. Deposit	:	Present or absent
4. Surface pellicle	:	Present or absent
5. Odour	:	Absent or fishy/earthy
6. Pigment	:	Pigmented/non-pigmented
7. Motility (after 2 hours of incubation)	:	Motile or non-motile

_____
Signature of Teacher

Gram Staining

Aim: To describe the morphological features of bacteria on Gram staining.

Morphological Characteristics of Bacteria on Gram Stain

1. Gram's reaction : Gram-positive or gram-negative
2. Shape   : Cocci: Spherical/oval/lanceolate/kidney shaped. Bacilli: Short/long rods, commas; spirals, cocco-bacilli.
3. Staining   : Uniform stainting/gram variable
4. Axis   : Straight/curved/spiral
5. Size   : Length and breadth (approx. in microns)
6. Sides   : Parallel, irregular
7. Ends   : Rounded, bulging, concave or pointed
8. Arrangement : Singly, in pairs, in chains, in tetrads, in clusters, thumb print, fish in stream, etc.

Constituents

1. Primary stain — crystal violet
2. Mordant   — iodine
3. Decolorizer   — acetone
4. Counterstain — Safranin

Principle of Gram Stain

The structure of the organism's cell wall determines whether the organism is gram positive or negative. When stained with a primary stain (e.g. crystal violet) and fixed by a mordant (iodine), some bacteria are able to retain the primary stain and resist decolorization (due to the presence of a thick petidoglycan layer—90% of cell wall) while gram negative bacteria have a thin peptidoglycan layer that allows primary stain to wash out by decolorizer and get counterstained (safranin). Thus gram-positive organisms stain purple and gram-negative organisms stain pink in color.

_____
Signature of Teacher

Staphylococcus aureus

Gram-positive cocci are seen in clusters

Staphylococcus aureus

Aim: To study the colony characteristics of *S. aureus* in the media provided and preparation of smear and Gram staining from the culture plate and study motilty from the broth provided.

Colony Characteristics of *Staphylococcus aureus*

1. Name of the media	:	Blood agar
2. Shape	:	Circular
3. Size	:	Pin head (2–4 mm)
4. Elevation	:	Raised, convex
5. Surface	:	Smooth, glistening
6. Edge	:	Entire
7. Opacity	:	White opaque
8. Consistency	:	Butyrous
9. Emulsifiability	:	Easy
10. Pigment	:	Golden yellow pigment present
11. Change in medium	:	Beta hemolysis present

Preparation of Smear for Gram Staining

- Take a clean grease free slide.
- Put a drop of normal saline in the middle of the glass slide.
- Sterilize a bacteriological loop by red hot flaming, allow to cool.
- Touch one colony of *Staphylococcus aureus* from the plate of blood agar provided.
- Emulsify the colony in the normal saline on the slide.
- Allow to air dry.
- Heat fix the slide by passing the glass slide with the smear 3–4 times across the flame.

Steps of Gram Staining

1. Pour **crystal violet (primary stain)** on the smear and keep for 1 min.
2. Decant the stain and pour **Gram's iodine (mordant)** on the smear.
3. Decant the iodine and **decolorize with acetone** for 2–3 seconds.
4. Wash the slide.
5. **Counterstain with safranin** for 1 min.

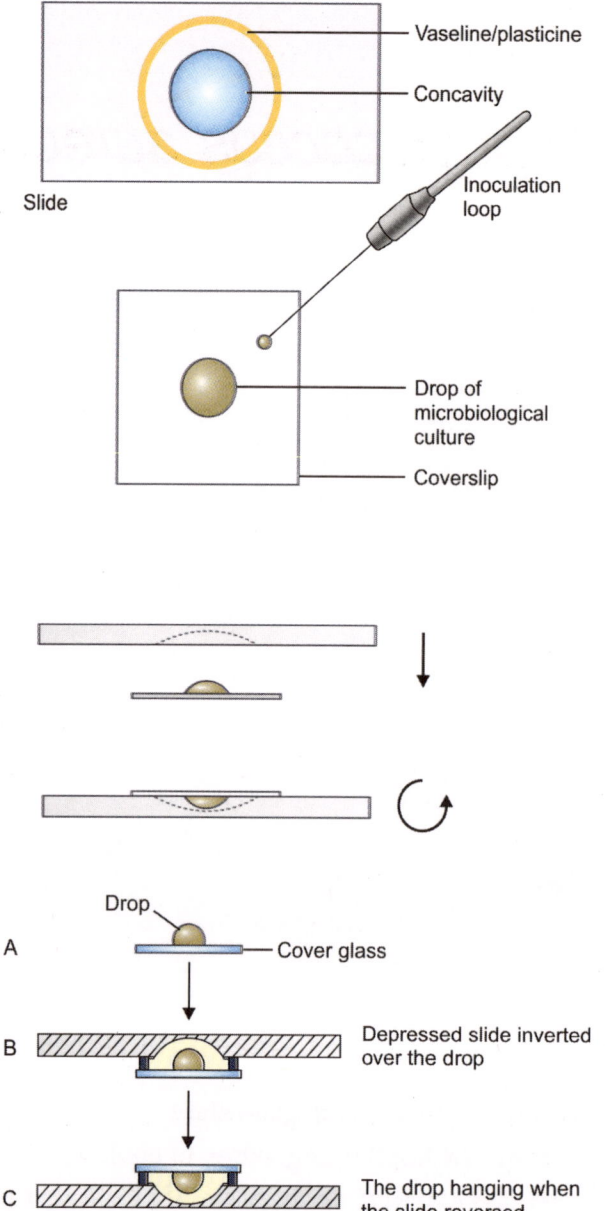

Hanging drop technique for bacterial motility examination

6. Wash the slide with water and air dry.

7. Focus the slide under the oil-imersion objective (100X) of a light microscope.

8. Observe and note your finding.

Observation

Gram-positive (violet colored) cocci are seen in grape like clusters.

Motility Preparation

- Take a loopful of the broth provided and place the drop on a coverslip.
- Invert a glass slide with a ring of plasticine on the coverslip.
- Turn the slide with coverslip facing upwards down so that the drop now hangs from the coverslip.
- Focus the edge of the drop under 10X objective of light microscope.
- Look at the movement of cocci or bacilli with respect to Brownian motion at 40X objective.
- Record your findings.

Observation of Motility of *Staphylococcus aureus* from the Broth Provided

Non-motile cocci are seen.

Confirmatory Tests for *Staphylococcus aureus*

1. Catalase test—positive
2. Coagulase test—positive

COAGULASE TEST

Slide Coagulase Test

- A milky emulsion in normal saline is prepared from isolated colony of *Staphylococcus aureus* on a clean glass slide.
- One loopful of sterile rabbit plasma is added to this emulsion and mixed thoroughly.
- The slide is then rocked to and fro.
- Visible clumps are formed if the test organism is *Staphylococcus aureus*.
- This is a test for identifying the "clumping factor" or bound coagulase.

Tube Coagulase Test

- 1:6 dilution of rabbit plasma in normal saline is prepared.
- 1 ml of this solution is taken in each of four test tubes.
- To each of the first three tubes one colony of the test strain, a known coagulase positive *S. aureus* and a known coagulase negative *strain of Staphylococcus* spp. are added respectively.
- The fourth is left as it is as a control.

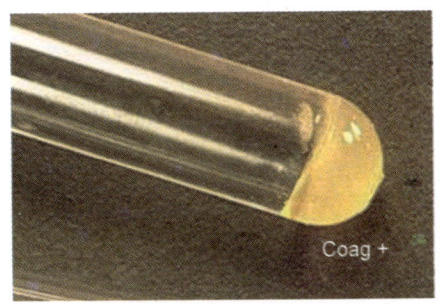

Staphylococcus aureus

Coag +

Tube coagulase test

Difference between *Staphylococcus* and *Micrococcus*		
Criteria	*Staphylococcus*	*Micrococcus*
Anaerobic growth	+	–
Carbohydrate utilization	Fermentative	Oxidative
Catalase	+	+
Oxidase (modified)	–	+
Bacitracin (0.04 U) disc	Resistant	Sensitive
Lysostaphin	Sensitive	Resistant
Difference between *Staphylococcus aureus* and *Staphylococcus epidermidis*		
Criteria	*Staphylococcus aureus*	*Staphylococcus epidermidis*
Pigment	+	–
Coagulase	+	–
Phosphatase	+	+
Mannitol fermentation	+	–
Trehalose fermentation	+	–
Difference between *Staphylococcus aureus* and *Staphylococcus saprophyticus*		
Criteria	*Staphylococcus aureus*	*Staphylococcus saprophyticus*
Pigment	+	V
Coagulase	+	–
Phosphatase	+	–
Mannitol fermentation	+	+
Novobiocin resistance	–	+

- The tubes are then incubated at 37°C and checked for clot formation every 30 minutes for up to 4 hours.
- Visible clot formation signifies production of coagulase enzyme and identifies the test strain as *S. aureus*.

Demonstration

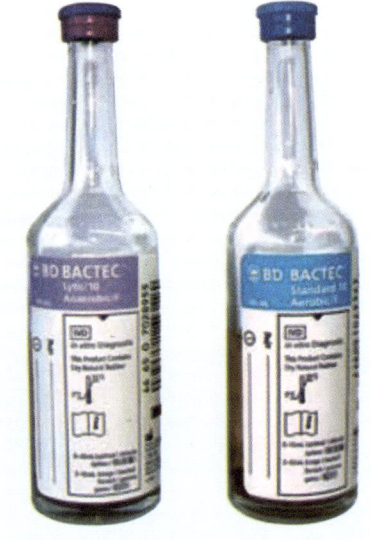

Automated blood culture bottles

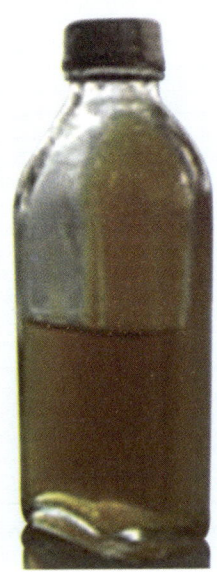

Biphasic blood culture bottle

Signature of Teacher

Streptococcus pyogenes

Gram-positive cocci are seen in chains

Streptococcus pyogenes

Aim: To study colony characteristics of *Streptococcus pyogenes* from blood agar *and* preparation of smear for gram staining, and study motility from the provided broth.

Colony Characteristics of *Streptococcus pyogenes*

1. Name of the media : Blood agar

2. Shape   : Circular

3. Size   : Pinpoint, 0.5–1 mm

4. Elevation   : Low convex

5. Surface   : Smooth, glistening

6. Edge   : Entire

7. Opacity   : Semi-transparent

8. Consistency   : Butyrous

9. Emulsifiability   : Easy

10. Pigment   : None

11. Change in medium: Wide zone of beta hemolysis is present around the colonies.

Smear and Gram Staining

- Put a drop of normal saline in the middle of a clean grease free glass slide.
- Make a smear of the colony provided, dry and heat fix the slide.
- Pour **crystal violet (primary stain)** on the smear and keep for 1 min.
- Decant the stain and pour **Gram's iodine (mordant)** on the smear.
- **Decolorize with acetone** for 2–3 seconds.
- Wash the slide and **counterstain with safranin** for 1 min.

Observation from Gram Staining of *Streptococcus pyogenes*

Gram-positive (violet colored) cocci are seen in short chains.

Observation of Motility of *Streptococcus pyogenes* from the Broth Provided

Non-motile cocci are seen.

Confirmatory Tests for *Streptococcus pyogenes*

1. Catalase test—negative

2. Sensitive to bacitracin disc (0.04 U)

3. CAMP test negative

4. Lancefield grouping by carbohydrate extraction method

Demonstration

- Gram stained smear of *Streptococcus pneumoniae* (pneumococci)
- Gram stained smear of enterococci spp.
- Candle jar

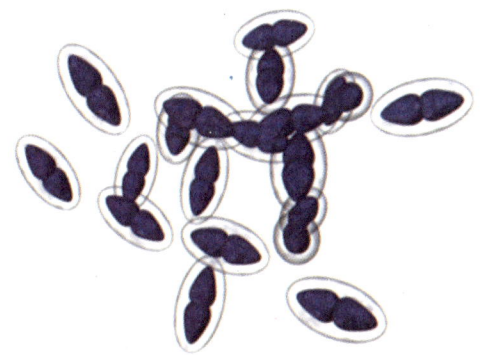

***Streptococcus pneumoniae* (pneumococci):** Gram-positive diplococci; Lanceolate/flame-shaped with wider ends adjacent.

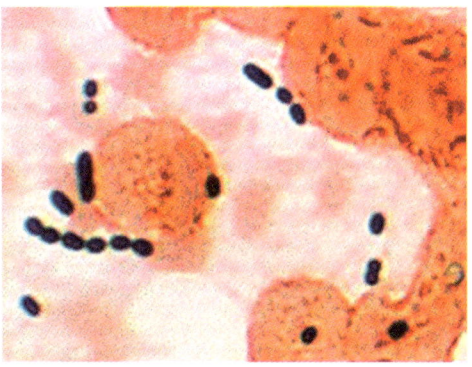

Enterococci: Gram-positive oval diplococci

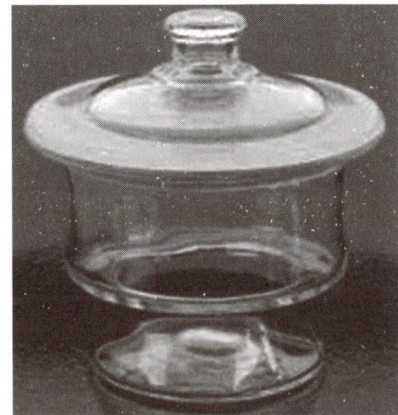

Candle jar: Used to provide capnophilic environment (5–10% CO_2) for the growth of certain organisms like *Streptococcus pneumoniae*. After keeping the inoculated plates, the candle inside is lighted and the lid is closed → cutting of external oxygen → extinguishes candle → relative increase (5–10%) of CO_2 inside the jar.

Signature of Teacher

Gram-Negative Cocci

Aim: To study the Gram stain characteristics of gram-negative diplococci:
1. *Neisseria gonorrhoeae*
2. *Neisseria meningitides*

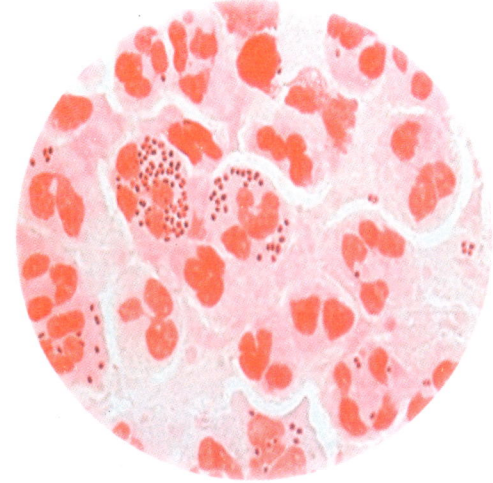

Intracellular gram-negative diplococci from uretheral discgarge (*Neisseria gonorrhoeae*)

Chocolate Agar

It is an enriched media for growth of
- *Neisseria* spp.
- Pneumococci
- *Haemophilus* spp.

Preparation of Chocolate Agar

Blood agar kept at 55°C for 1 hour becomes chocolate agar due to lysis of RBCs.

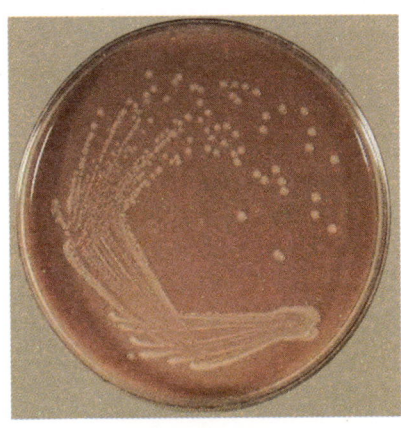

Chocolate agar

Signature of Teacher

Culture Media and Biochemical Reactions of Enterobacteriaceae Family

The following media are commonly used for gram-negative bacilli of the family Enterobacteriaceae.

Blood Agar

- It is an **enriched medium.**
- Contains **5% sheep blood** in nutrient agar.
- Helps to differentiate between **α and β hemolysis.**
- Helps to **study swarming** by *Proteus* spp.
- Preparation: Autoclaved nutrient agar is cooled to 50°C followed by addition of defibrinated sheep blood aseptically.

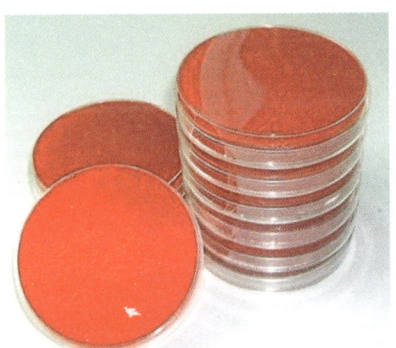 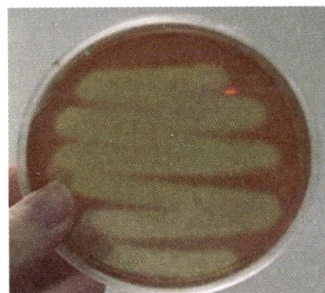 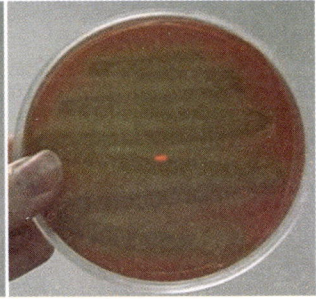

Beta hemolysis   Alpha hemolysis

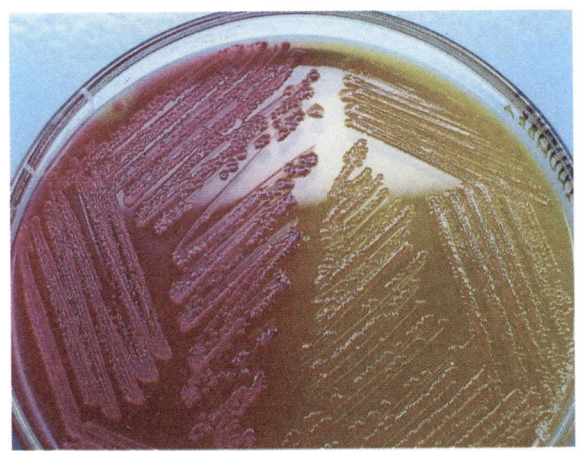

Lactose fermentor colonies   Non-lactose fermentor colonies

MacCankey agar

MacConkey Agar

- It is a **mildly selective media** as it selects out lactose fermenting (**LF) pink colonies** from non-lactose fermenting (**NLF) pale colonies**.
- It is also an **indicator medium** and contains neutral red indicator
- Contains bile salt (sodium taurocholate) hence **prevents swarming.**

Xylose Lysine Deoxycholate (XLD) Agar

Moderately selective media for
- *Salmonella* (pink colonies with black centre)
- *Shigella* (pink colonies)

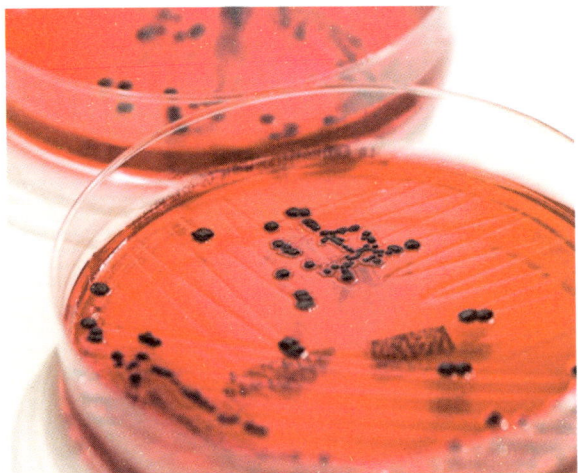

XLD agar

BIOCHEMICAL TESTS

Catalase Test

Principle: Many bacteria produce catalase enzyme which breaks down H_2O_2 into water and oxygen. This enzyme produces immediate bubble formation (due to oxygen production), when the growth of the organism is added to a drop of 3% H_2O_2 on a slide.

Examples: Positive—*Staphylococcus*; members of Enterobacteriaceae family
Negative—*Streptococcus* spp.

Oxidase Test

Reagent: Tetramethyl *para*-phenylenediamine dihydrochloride

Test:
- A strip impregnated with the reagent is taken.
- A small portion of the colony is picked-up with the corner of a sterile coverslip and smeared onto the strip.
- Change of color to purple within 30 sec signifies positive reaction.

Principle: The cytrochrome oxidase enzyme of certain bacteria is able to oxidize the reagent producing the coloured product.

Example: Positive—*Pseudomomas* spp., *Vibrio* spp.
Negative—members of family Enterobacteriaceae

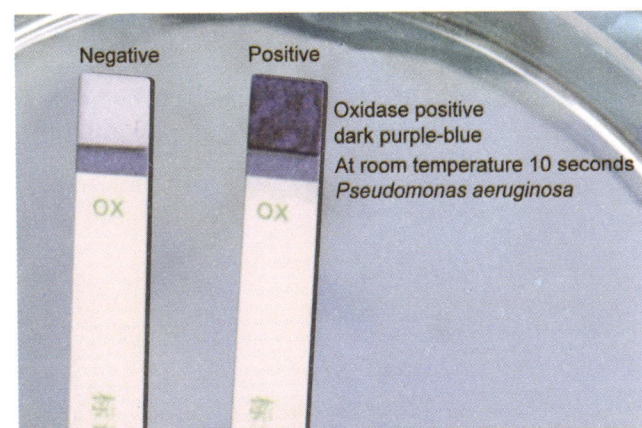

Oxidase test

Indole Production Test

- **Principle of test:** Ability of an organisn to split indole from tryptophan.
- **Reagent used:** Kovac's reagent
- Indole producing organisms: *E. coli, Proteus vulgaris*.

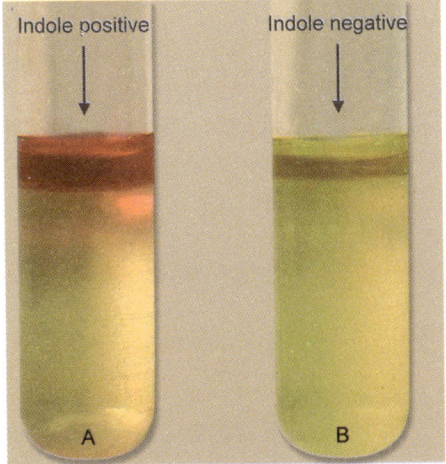

Indole production test

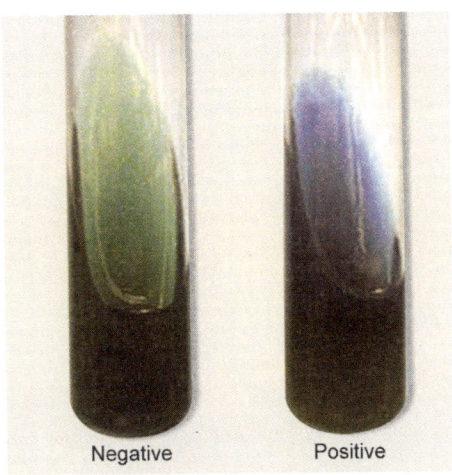

Citrate utilization test

Citrate Utilization Test

- **Principle:** Ability of an organism to utilize citrate as the sole source of carbon for metabolism resulting in alkalinity.
- **Medium:** Simmon's citrate medium
- **Indicator:** Bromothymol blue
- **Citrate utilizing organisms:** *Klebsiella, Salmonella, Enterobacter*

Urease Production Test

- **Principle:** Ability of an organism to produce the enzyme urease which hydrolyze urea to ammonia resulting in pink color.
- **Medium:** Christensen's urea agar
- **Indicator:** Phenol red
- Urease producing organisms: *Proteus, Providencia, Helicobacter pylori, Klebsiella, Cryptococcus* (yeast fungus)

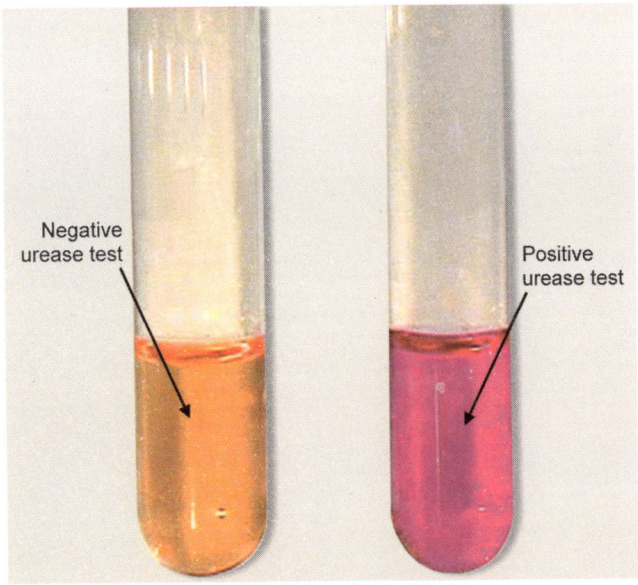

Urease production test

Methyl Red (MR) Test

- **Principle:** Ability of an organism to produce and maintain stable acid end-products from glucose fermentation and overcome buffering capacity of the system.
- **Medium:** Glucose phosphate broth
- **MR positive organisms:** *E. coli*, *Yersinia* spp.

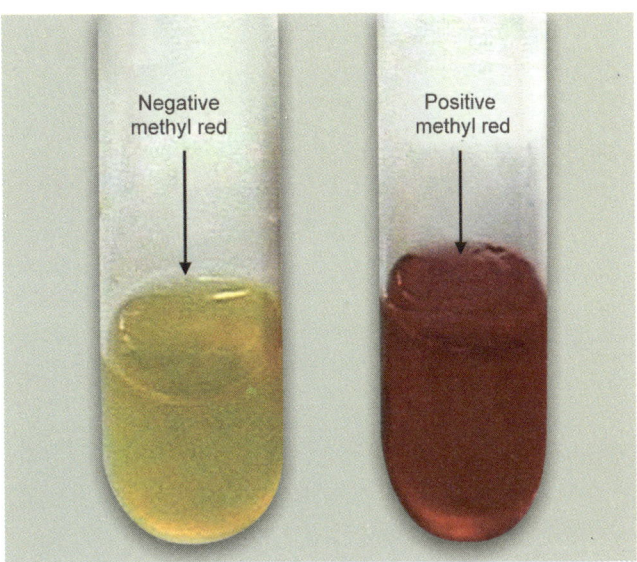

Methyl red test

Voges-Proskauer (VP) Test

- **Principle:** Ability of an organism to produce neutral end product acetylmethyl carbinol/acetoin from glucose fermentation
- **Medium:** Glucose phosphate broth
- **VP positive organisms:** *Klebsiella*, *Enterobacter*

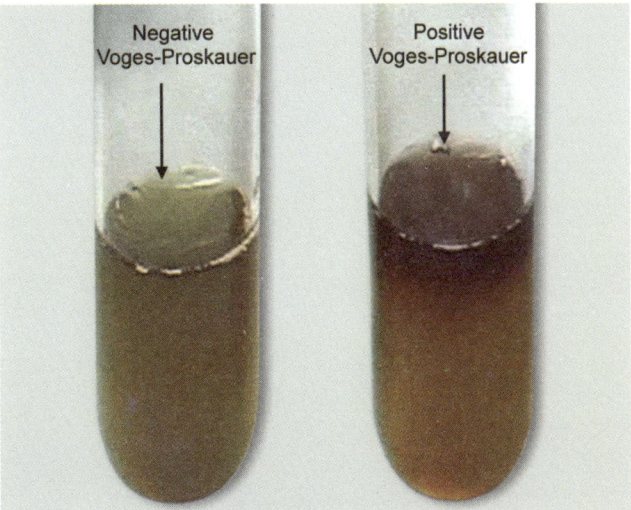

Voges-Proskauer test

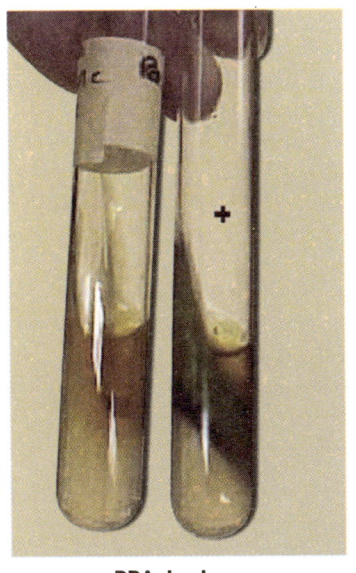

PPA test

Phenylalanine Deaminase (PPA) Test

- **Principle:** Ability of an organism to deaminate phenylalanine to phenyl pyruvic acid (PPA) by enzyme deaminase leading to acidity.
- Addition of 10% $FeCl_3$ leads to production of green colored compound.
- PPA positive organisms:
  - *Proteus* spp.
  - *Providencia* spp.

H₂S Production Test

- **Principle:** Ability of an organism to liberate H_2S from sulphur bearing amino acids leading to production of a visible black color reaction.
- **Indicator:** Ferric ammonium citrate/lead acetate
- **H₂S positive organisms:** *Salmonella typhi, Citrobacter freundii, Edwardsiella* spp.

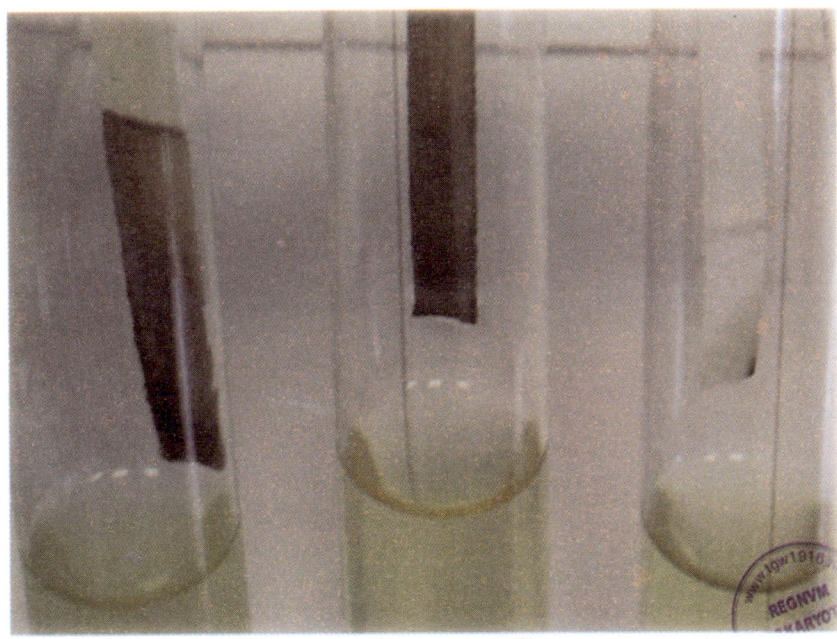

H₂S production test

Nitrate Reduction Test

Principle: Ability of an organism to produce nitrate reductase enzyme that reduces nitrate to nitrite which results in production of a red color when equal volumes of sulphanilic acid and alpha naphthylamine are added to an overnight growth of the organism in nitrate broth.

Nitrate Reduction Test Positive Organisms

- All organisms of the Enterobacteriaceae family
- *Vibrio cholerae*
- *Pseudomonas aeruginosa*

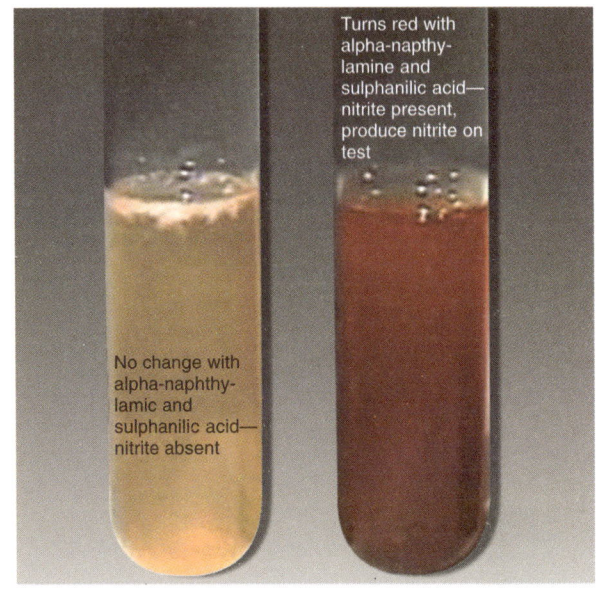

Turns red with alpha-napthylamine and sulphanilic acid—nitrite present, produce nitrite on test

No change with alpha-naphthylamic and sulphanilic acid—nitrite absent

Nitrate reduction test

Oxidation Fermentation (OF) Test

Principle: To determine whether certain gram-negative bacilli metabolize glucose by fermentation or aerobic respiration (oxidatively). During the anaerobic process of fermentation, pyruvate is converted to a variety of mixed acids depending on the type of fermentation. The high concentration of acid produced during fermentation will **OF media (Hugh and Leifson media)** in the presence or absence of oxygen .

Certain non-fermenting gram-negative bacteria metabolize glucose using aerobic respiration and therefore only produce a small amount of weak acids during glycolysis and Krebs cycle. The decreased amount of peptone and increased amount of glucose facilitate the detection of weak acids thus produced.

Uses: OF test is used to determine if gram-negative bacteria metabolize carbohydrates oxidatively or fermentatively.

- Oxidative, e.g. *Pseudomonas*
- Fermentative, e.g. organisms of family Enterobacteriaceae, *Vibrio*
- Non-sacchrolytic (have no ability to use the carbohydrate in the media), e.g. *Alkaligenes fecalis*

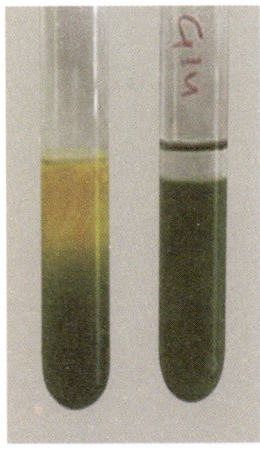

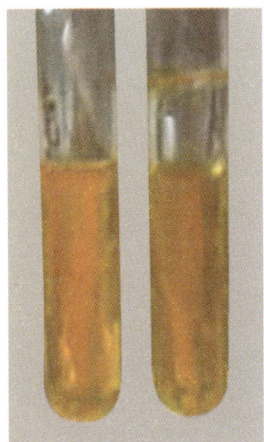

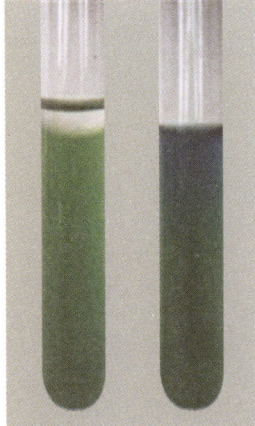

Oxidative   **Fermentative**   **Non-sacchrolytic**   Signature of Teacher

Escherichia coli

Long thin gram-nagative bacilli are seen

Escherichia coli

Aim: To study the colony characteristics *of Escherichia coli* from MacConkey agar, preparation of smear and Gram staining, and study motility from the provided broth.

Colony Characteristics of *Escherichia coli*

1. Name of the media : MacConkey agar
2. Shape : Circular
3. Size : Small to large
4. Elevation : Flat
5. Surface : Smooth, glistening
6. Edge : Entire
7. Opacity : Opaque/partially translucent
8. Emulsifiability : Easy
9. Pigment : None
10. Change in medium : Pink due to lactose fermentation

Smear and Gram Staining

- Put a drop of normal saline in the middle of a clean grease free glass slide.
- Make a smear of the colony provided, dry and heat fix the slide.
- Pour **crystal violet (primary stain)** on the smear and keep for 1 min.
- Decant the stain and pour **Gram's iodine (mordant)** on the smear.
- **Decolourize with acetone** for 2–3 seconds.
- Wash the slide and **counterstain with safranin** for 1 min.

Observation of Gram Staining of *Escherichia coli*

Gram-negative long straight bacilli with parallel sides and pointed ends are seen.

Observation of Motility of *Escherichia coli* from the Broth Provided

Motile bacilli are seen.

Confirmatory Tests for *Escherichia coli*

1. Catalase test—positive; Oxidase test—negative.
2. Glucose and lactose are fermented with production of acid and gas.
3. Nitrate is reduced to nitrite.
4. Fermentative utilization of sugars in OF media.
5. Indole production and methyl red tests are positive.
6. VP and citrate tests are negative.

_____
Signature of Teacher

Klebsiella spp.

Short plump gram-nagative bacilli are seen

Klebsiella

Aim: To study colony characteristics of *Klebsiella* from MacConkey agar, preparation of smear and Gram staining, and study motility from the provided broth.

Colony Characteristics of *Klebsiella* spp.

1. Name of the media : MacConkey agar
2. Shape : Circular
3. Size : Large
4. Elevation : Dome shaped
5. Surface : Smooth, glistening
6. Edge : Entire
7. Consistency : Mucoid
8. Emulsifiability : Easy
9. Pigment : None
10. Change in medium : Pink due to fermentation of lactose

Smear and Gram Staining

- Put a drop of normal saline in the middle of a clean grease free glass slide.
- Make a smear of the colony provided, dry and heat fix the slide.
- Pour **crystal violet (primary stain)** on the smear and keep for 1 min.
- Decant the stain and pour **Gram's iodine (mordant)** on the smear.
- **Decolorize with acetone** for 2–3 seconds.
- Wash the slide and **counterstain with safranin** for 1 min.

Observation of Gram Staining of *Klebsiella* spp.

Short plump straight gram negative bacilli are seen.

Observation of Motility of *Klebsiella* spp. from the Broth Provided

Non-motile bacilli are seen.

Confirmatory Tests for *Klebsiella* spp.

1. Catalase test—positive; Oxidase test—negative.
2. Glucose and lactose are fermented with production of acid and gas.
3. Nitrate is reduced to nitrite.
4. Fermentative utilization of sugars in OF media.
5. Indole production and methyl red tests are negative.
6. VP and citrate tests are positive

Common species: *K. pneumoniae, K. oxytoca.*

Signature of Teacher

Proteus spp.

Gram-nagative bacilli are seen

Proteus

Aim: To study colony characteristics of **Proteus** from blood agar, preparation of smear and Gram staining, and study motility from the provided broth.

Colony Characteristics of *Proteus* spp.

- Swarming growth of *Proteus* is seen on blood agar.
- Seminal/fishy odour is appreciated.
- On MacConkey agar, grows as pale non-lactose fermenting (NLF) colonies with typical fishy odour.

Smear and Gram Staining

- Put a drop of normal saline in the middle of a clean grease free glass slide.
- Make a smear of the colony provided, dry and heat fix the slide.
- Pour **crystal violet (primary stain)** on the smear and keep for 1 min.
- Decant the stain and pour **Gram's iodine (mordant)** on the smear.
- **Decolorize with acetone** for 2–3 seconds.
- Wash the slide and **counterstain with safranin** for 1 min.

Observation of Gram Staining of *Proteus* spp.

Gram-negative bacilli are seen.

Observation of Motility of *Proteus* from the Broth Provided

Motile bacilli are seen.

Confirmatory Tests for *Proteus* spp.

1. Catalase test—positive; Oxidase test—negative.
2. Glucose is fermented with production of acid and gas.
3. Lactose is not fermented.
4. Nitrate is reduced to nitrite.
5. Fermentative utilization of sugars in OF media.
6. Urease test—positive; PPA test—positive; H_2S is produced.
7. Indole production test is negative (except *P. vulgaris*).
8. Citrate test is negative.

Common species: *P. mirabilis, P. vulgaris.*

_____
Signature of Teacher

Salmonella spp.

Gram-nagative bacilli are seen

Salmonella

Aim: To study colony characteristics of *Salmonella* from MacConkey agar, preparation of smear and Gram staining, and study motility from the provided broth.

Colony Characteristics of *Salmonella* spp.

Non-lactose fermenting (NLF) colonies (pale) are seen.

1. Name of the media : MacConkey agar
2. Shape : Circular
3. Size : Large 1–3 μm × 0.5 μm
4. Elevation : Low convex
5. Surface : Smooth
6. Edge : Irregular
7. Opacity : Translucent
8. Pigment : None
9. Change in medium : No change due to non-fermentation of lactose
10. Odour : None

Smear and Gram Staining

- Put a drop of normal saline in the middle of a clean grease free glass slide.
- Make a smear of the colony provided, dry and heat fix the slide.
- Pour **crystal violet (primary stain)** on the smear and keep for 1 min.
- Decant the stain and pour **Gram's iodine (mordant)** on the smear.
- **Decolorize with acetone** for 2–3 seconds.
- Wash the slide and **counterstain with safranin** for 1 min.

Observation of Gram Staining of *Salmonella* spp.

Gram-negative bacilli are seen.

Observation of Motility of *Salmonella* from the Broth Provided

Motile bacilli are seen.

Confirmatory Tests for *Salmonella* spp.

1. Catalase test—positive
2. Oxidase test—negative

3. Glucose is fermented with production of acid and gas (except *S. typhi*).

4. Lactose is not fermented.

5. Nitrate is reduced to nitrite.

6. Fermentative utilization test of sugars in OF media.

7. H_2S is produced.

8. MR test—positive; VP test—negative

9. Citrate test—positive

10. Urease test, indole production test—negative

11. Confirmation by *serotyping*.

Demonstration

- Growth characteristic of *Salmonella typhi* on XLD agar and Wilson and Blair bismuth sulphite media.
- Widal test.
- Craigies tube is used for phase conversion of *Salmonalla* serotypes.

Wilson and Blair Bisthmuth Sulphite Media

- Highly selective media for *Salmonella typhi*
- Jet black colonies with a metallic sheen are formed due to reduction of tellurite to metallic tellurium.

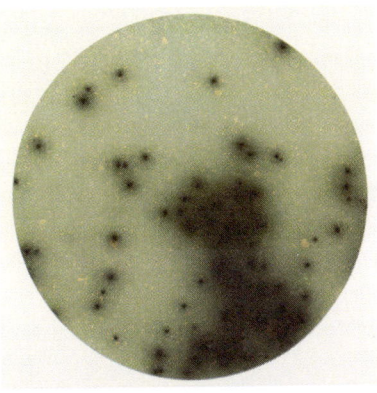

Salmonella typhi in Wilson and Blair bismuth sulphite media

Xylose Lysine Deoxycholate Agar (XLD Agar)

Pink colonies with black centre are seen suggestive of *Salmonella* spp.

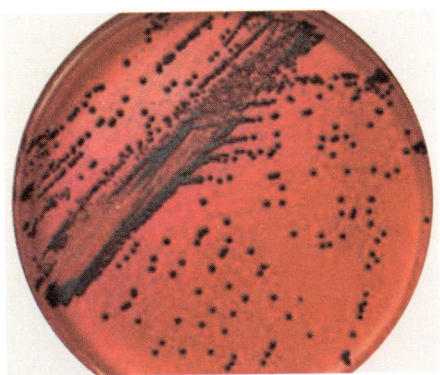

Salmonella in XLD agar

Serological Test for Enteric Fever: Serum helps in antibody formation.

Widal Test

Principle: This is a **tube agglutination test** for the diagnosis of enteric fever. The titre of antibodies in the patient's serum is determined by the agglutination of particulate *Salmonella* antigen.

Antigens Used in the Test

- "O" antigen of *Salmonella typhi*
- "H" antigen of *Salmonella typhi*
- "H" antigen of *Salmonella paratyphi* A
- "H" antigen of *Salmonella paratyphi* B
  ("O" antigen is shared among the species.)

Agglutination

- "O" agglutination—compact chalky granular deposit
- "H" agglutination—loose, fluffy or cotton wooly deposit

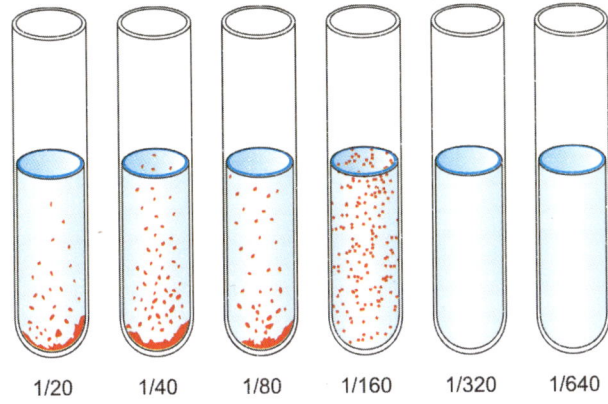

| 1/20 | 1/40 | 1/80 | 1/160 | 1/320 | 1/640 |

Craigies tube is used for phase conversion of *Salmonalla* serotypes.

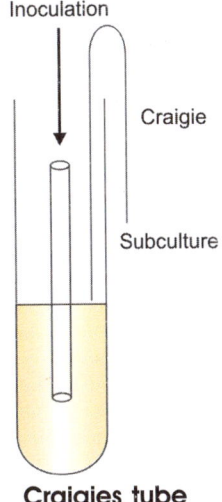

Craigies tube

Signature of Teacher

Shigella spp.

Gram-nagative bacilli are seen

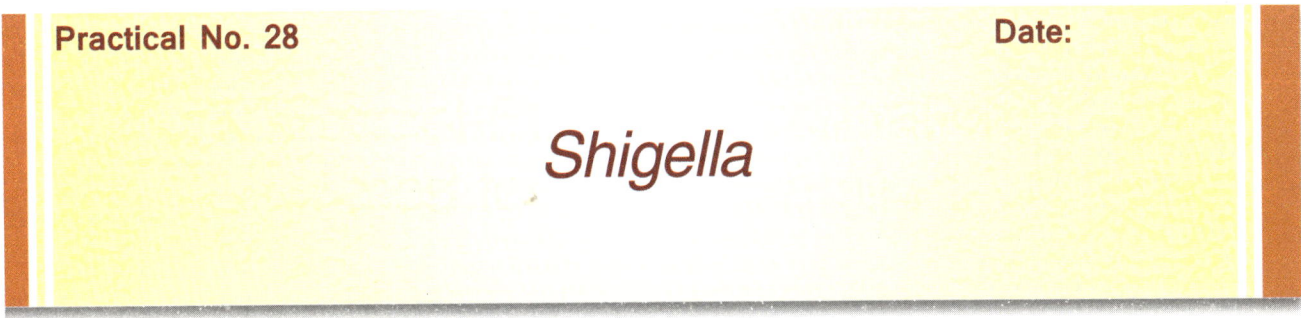

Shigella

Aim: To study colony characteristics of *Shigella* from MacConkey agar, preparation of smear and Gram staining, and study motility from the provided broth.

Colony Characteristics of *Shigella* spp.

NLF colonies are seen.

1. Name of the media	:	MacConkey agar
2. Shape	:	Circular
3. Size	:	Small 2 mm
4. Elevation	:	Flat
5. Surface	:	Smooth, glistening
6. Opacity	:	Translucent
7. Consistency	:	Smooth
8. Emulsifiability	:	Easy
9. Pigment	:	None
10. Change in medium	:	No change due to non-fermentation of lactose

Smear and Gram Staining

- Put a drop of normal saline in the middle of a clean grease free glass slide.
- Make a smear of the colony provided, dry and heat fix the slide.
- Pour **crystal violet (primary stain)** on the smear and keep for 1 min.
- Decant the stain and pour **Gram's iodine (mordant)** on the smear.
- **Decolorize with acetone** for 2–3 seconds.
- Wash the slide and **counterstain with safranin** for 1 min.

Observation from Gram Staining of *Shigella* spp.

Gram-negative bacilli are seen.

Observation of Motility of *Shigella* spp. from the Broth Provided

Non-motile bacilli are seen.

Confirmatory Tests for *Shigella* spp.

1. Catalase test—positive
2. Oxidase test—negative
3. Glucose is fermented with production of acid without gas.
4. Nitrate is reduced to nitrite.
5. Fermentative utilization of sugars in of media.
6. MR test—positive; VP test—negative
7. Citrate test—positive
8. Urease test, indole production test—negative
9. Confirmation by *serotyping*.

Biochemical Reactions of *Shigella* species

Biochemical tests	*Shigella* species			
	S. dysenteriae	*S. flexneri*	*S. boydii*	*S. sonnei*
Glucose	Only acid, no gas	Only acid, no gas	Only acid, no gas	Only acid, no gas
Lactose	–	–	–	Late lactose fermenter
Sucrose	–	–	–	–
Maltose	–	–	–	–
Mannitol	–	Acid	Acid	Acid
Indole	Variable	Variable	Variable	Variable
Methyl red	+	+	+	+
VP	–	–	–	–
Urease	–	–	–	–
Ornithine decarboxylase	–	–	–	+
Lysine decarboxylase	–	–	–	–

Signature of Teacher

Pseudomonas spp.

Gram-nagative bacilli are seen

Non-Fermenters: *Pseudomonas*

Aim: To study colony characteristics of ***Pseudomonas*** spp. from nutrient agar, preparation of smear and Gram staining, and study motility from the provided broth.

Colony Characteristics of *Pseudomonas*

1. Name of the media   : Nutrient agar
2. Shape   : Circular
3. Size   : Large
4. Elevation   : Flat
5. Surface   : Smooth, glistening with a metallic sheen
6. Edge   : Irregular
7. Consistency   : Opaque
8. Emulsifiability   : Easy
9. Pigment   : Green colored diffusible pigments are seen.
10. Change in medium   : Green colored due to diffusible pigment
11. Odour   : Musty/earthy smell is appreciated

Non-lactose fermenting (NLF) colonies with characteristic musty/frooty odour are seen on MacConkey agar.

Smear and Gram Staining

- Put a drop of normal saline in the middle of a clean grease free glass slide.
- Make a smear of the colony provided, dry and heat fix the slide.
- Pour **crystal violet (primary stain)** on the smear and keep for 1 min.
- Decant the stain and pour **Gram's iodine (mordant)** on the smear.
- **Decolorize with acetone** for 2–3 seconds.
- Wash the slide and **counterstain with safranin** for 1 min.

Observation of Gram Stain of *Pseudomonas* spp.

Gram-negative bacilli are seen.

Common species: The most common species is *Pseudomonas aeruginosa*.

Observation of Motility of *Pseudomonas* spp. from the Broth Provided

Actively motile bacilli are seen.

Confirmatory Tests for *Pseudomonas* spp.

1. Catalase test—positive
2. Oxidase test—positive
3. Nitrate is reduced to nitrite.
4. Oxidative utilization of sugars in OF media.
5. Arginine dihydrolase test is positive.

Signature of Teacher

Practical No. 30   **Date:**

Demonstration of *Vibrio, Spirochaete* and *Chlamydia trachomatis*

Characteristics of *Vibrio Cholerae*

- Grows as non-lactose fermenters (NLF) on MacConkey agar.
- Grows as yellow sucrose fermenting colonies on thiosulphate citrate bile salt sucrose (TCBS) agar.
- Actively motile showing darting motility.

Demonstration

- TCBS
- Silver stained slide of *Spirochaeta, Leptospira.*
- Giemsa stained slide from irradiated MacCoy cells showing elementary bodies of *Chlamydia trachomatis.*

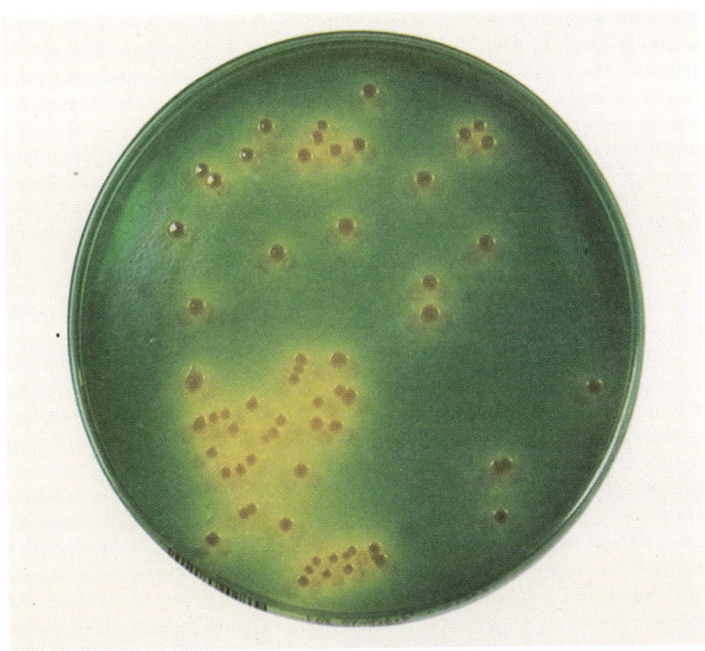

Thiosulphate citrate bilesalt sucrose (TCBS) media showing sucrose fermenting yellow colonies of *V. cholerae*

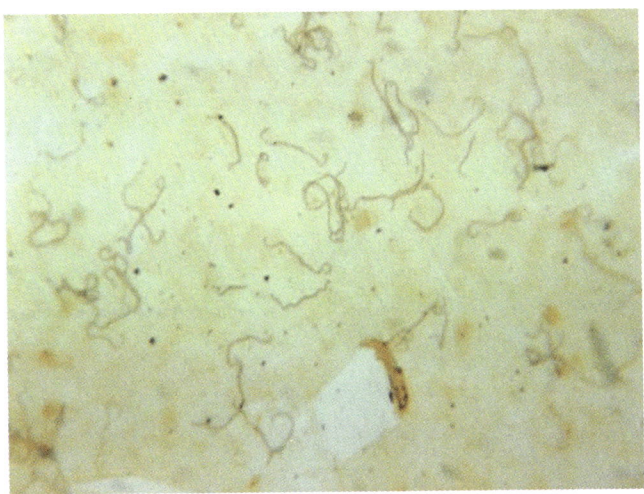

Slide of the *Spirochaeta, Leptospira* with umbrella hooked ends, stained by silver impregnation method (Fontanna's method)

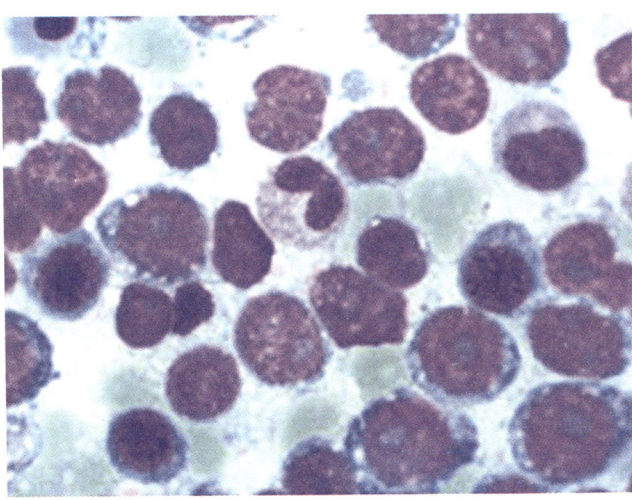

Giemsa stained slide from irradiated MacCoy cells showing elementary bodies of *Chlamydia trachomatis*

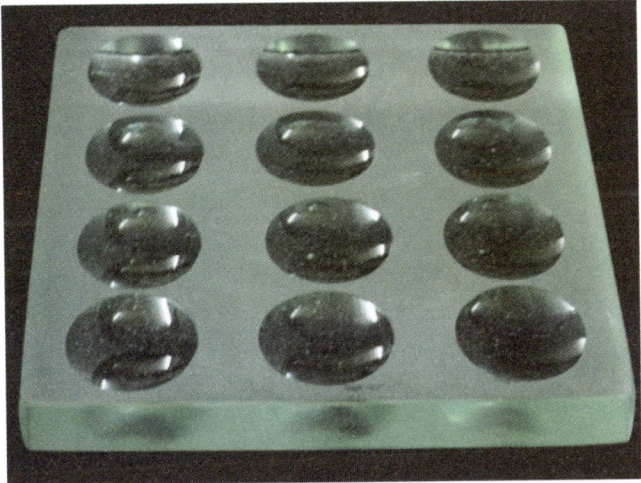

VDRL plate used for serological test of syphilis caused by *Treponema pallidum*

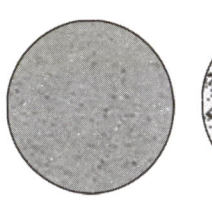 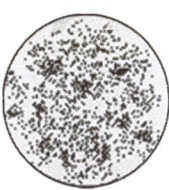 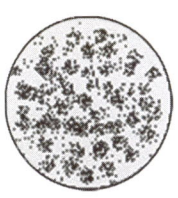

Non-reactive   Weakly reactive   Strongly reactive

VDRL reaction

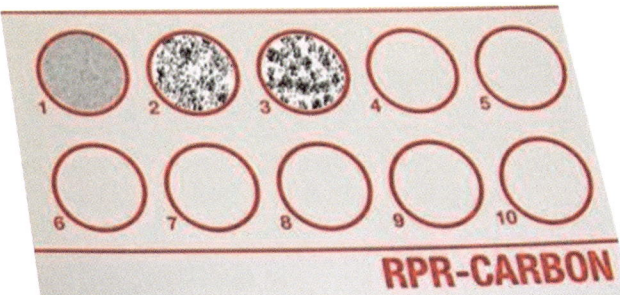

Rapid plasma regin (RPR) test for the diagnosis of syphilis

Signature of Teacher

Spore Staining and Anaerobic Methods

Aim: To study spore morphology by different staining methods.

Spore Staining by Modified Ziehn-Neelsen (ZN) Stain

1. Stain the smear after fixation with carbol fuchsin for 3–5 minutes heating the preparation until steam rises.
2. Wash in water.
3. Decolorize with 0.5% of H_2SO_4 for few minutes.
4. Wash with water.
5. Counterstain with 1% aqueous methylene blue for 2 minutes.
6. Wash with water and dry.
7. Focus under 100X objective of oil-immersion lens.

Observation: Spore stains bright red while protoplasm stains blue.

Spore Staining by Malachite Green Stain

1. Place slide over beaker of boiling water with bacterial film uppermost.
2. When large droplets condense on underside of slide, flood slide with 5% aqueous solution of malachite green for 1 minute while the water continues to boil.
3. Wash in cold water.
4. Add 0.5% safranin for 30 seconds.
5. Wash and dry.
6. Focus under 100X objective of oil-immersion lens.

Observation: Red spores inside green colored bacilli are seen.

Demonstration

- To study morphological characteristic features of *Clostridium tetani* from the stained smear provided.
- To identify the following: **MacIntosh and Field's anaerobic jar, gas pak system, Robertson's cooked meat broth, Thioglycollate broth** and know its uses.

Characteristic Features of *Clostridium tetani*

- **Obligatory anaerobic** bacterium
- **Gram-positive** bacilli
- **Spores: Spherical, terminal**, bulging
- Gram stain resembles **drumsticks**.
- **Habitat:** Found as spores in soil or in the gastrointestinal tract of animals.

  Disease caused: **Tetanus**

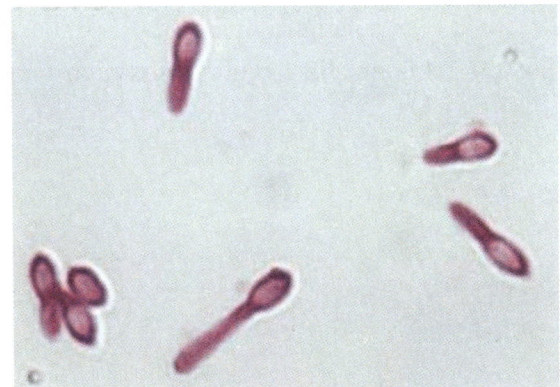

Clostridium tetani

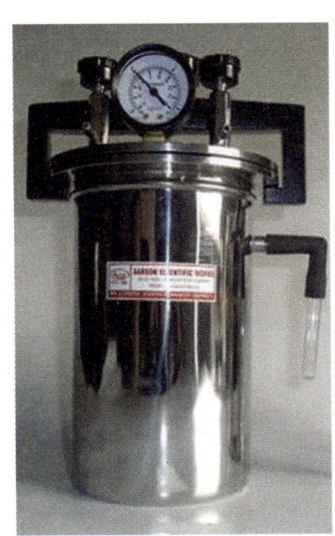

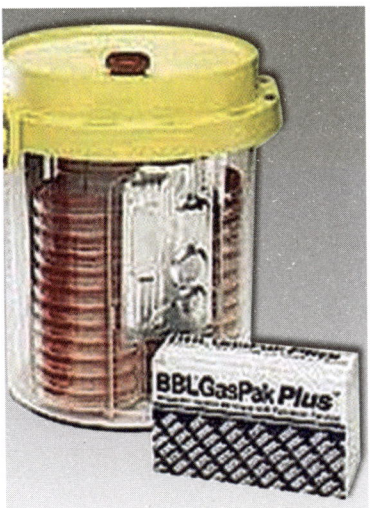

MacIntosh and Field's anaerobic jar

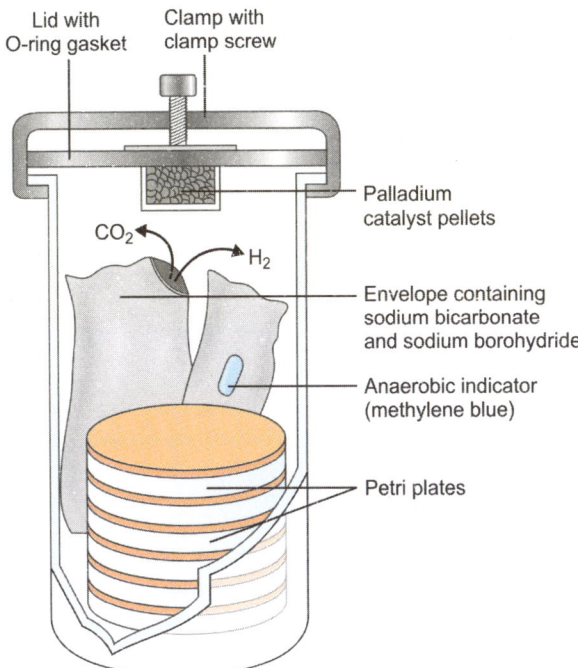

Lid with O-ring gasket

Clamp with clamp screw

Palladium catalyst pellets

CO_2

H_2

Envelope containing sodium bicarbonate and sodium borohydride

Anaerobic indicator (methylene blue)

Petri plates

GasPak system

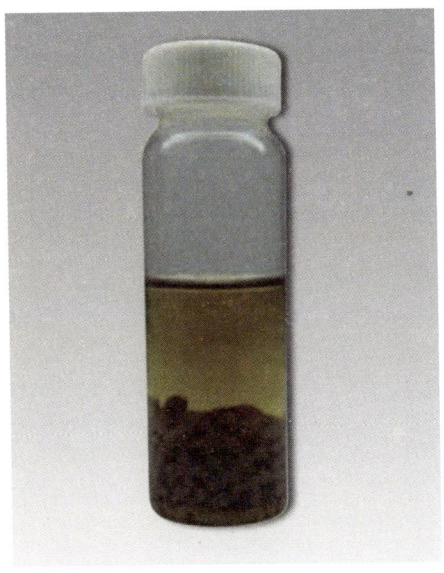

Robertson's cooked meat broth

Principle of RCM/CMB

- Robertson's cooked meat/cooked meat broth (RCM/CMB) contains fat free minced and cooked beef/ox heart (suspended in nutrient broth), the muscle protein that supplies amino acids and other nutrients.
- Unsaturated fatty acids present in meat utilize oxygen for auto-oxidation; this reaction is catalyzed by haematin in the meat.
- It also contains glutathione and cysteine (both are reducing agents) that enables the growth of obligate anaerobes by utilizing oxygen. Because reducing substances are more available in denatured protein, the meat particles are cooked before use in the medium.
- Sulphydryl compounds (present in cysteine) also contribute to the reducing effect.
- Growth in this medium is indicated by the turbidity.
- Blackening and decay of the meat particles indicate proteolysis.
- Before inoculation RCM/CMB medium is boiled to make it oxygen free. Allow the medium to cool to room temperature before inoculating it. The surface of CMB medium may be covered with a layer of sterile liquid paraffin to cut off oxygen supply.

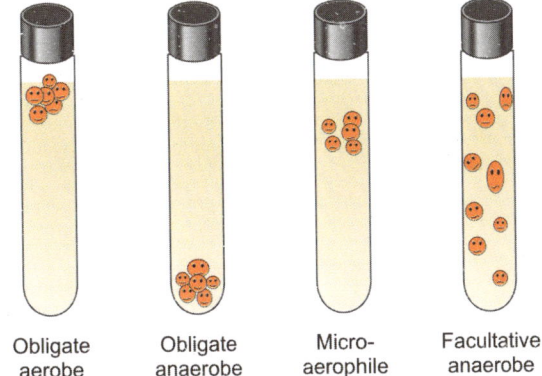

| Obligate aerobe | Obligate anaerobe | Micro-aerophile | Facultative anaerobe |

Thioglycollate broth contains nutrient broth and 1% thioglycollate for cultivation of anaerobes.

Signature of Teacher

Mycology Practical

32. Characteristic Features of Fungi

Characteristic Features of Fungi

Aim: To study morphological features of various fungi under microscope.

1. Yeast—*Candida* on Gram stained smear
2. Mould—*Aspergillus* spp., *Rhizopus* spp. and *Penicillium* spp. on lactophenol cotton blue (LPCB) mount

Gram Stained Smear of *Candida* spp.

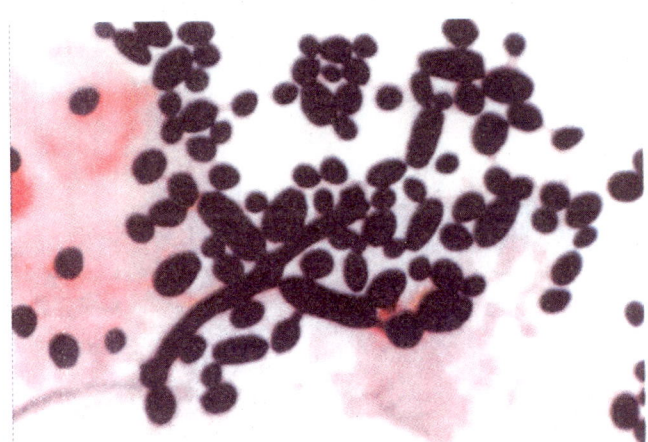

Showing gram-positive oval budding yeast cells

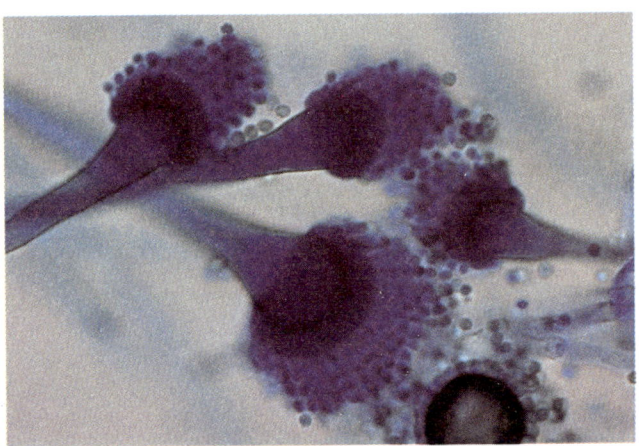

LPCB of *Aspergillus* spp.

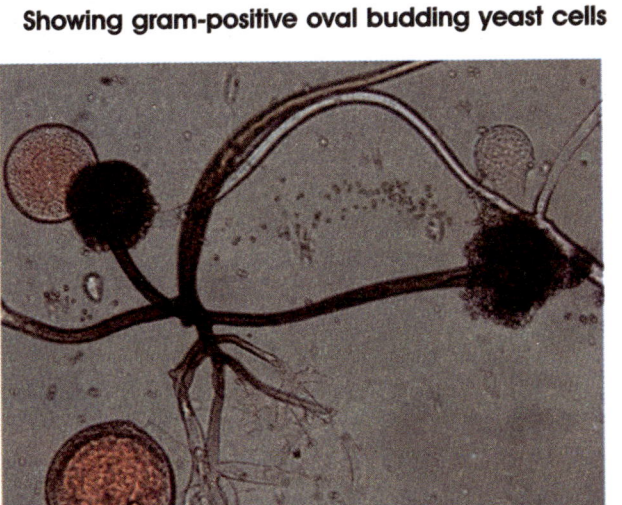

LPCB of *Rhizopus* spp.

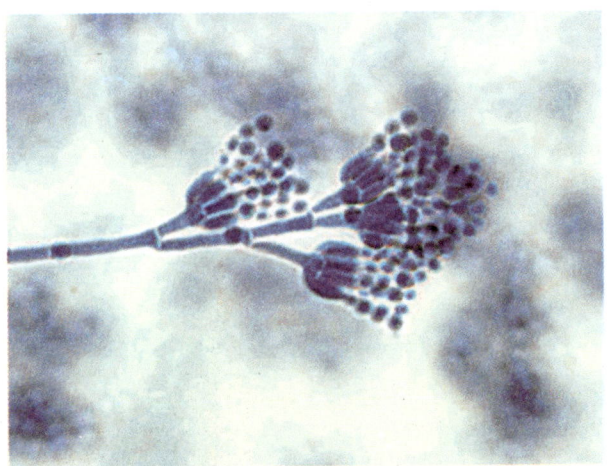

LPCB of *Penicillium* spp.

Slide Culture Set

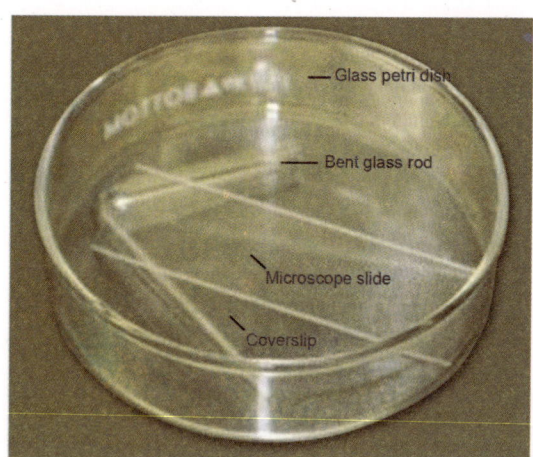

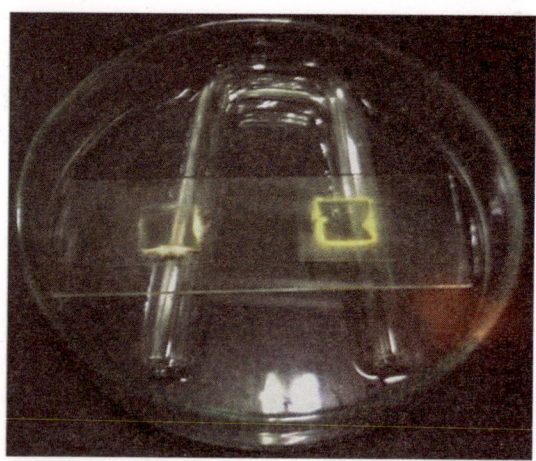

Slide Culture Components

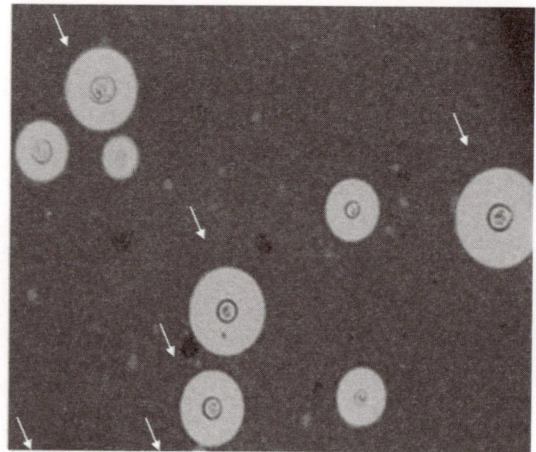

India ink preparation showing capsule of *Cryptococcus neoformans*

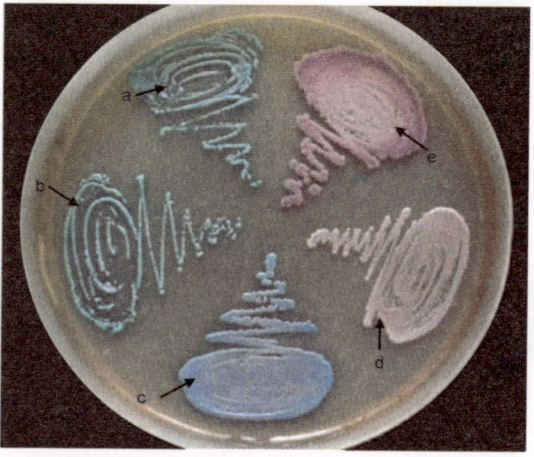

Chrome agar with growth of yeasts with different colours

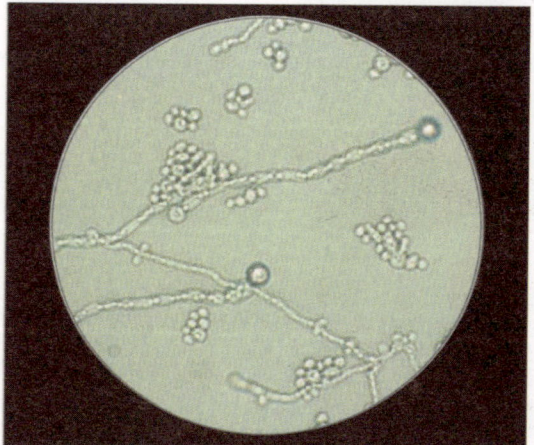

Corn meal agar showing terminal chlamydophores of *Candida albicans*

Demonstration

1. SDA (Sabouraud's dextrose agar)
2. Biphasic fungal blood culture media
3. SDA with growth of yeast
4. SDA with growth of mycelial fungi
5. Slide culture set
6. Chrome agar with growth of yeasts.
7. Corn meal agar
8. India ink preparation

Sabouraud's Dextrose Agar (SDA)

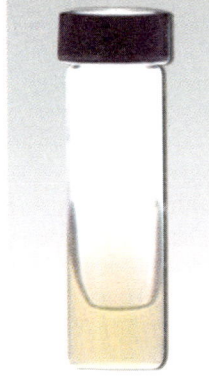

SDA

- With antibiotic (cap red cotton)
- Without antibiotic (cap white cotton).
- **Contains**
  - Dextrose—4%
  - Peptone—1%
  - pH—5–6
  - *Antibiotic chloramphenicol*—0.5 mg/ml (to prevent bacterial overgrowth)
  - *Cychloheximide*—0.005 mg/ml (to prevent growth of saprophytic fungus)

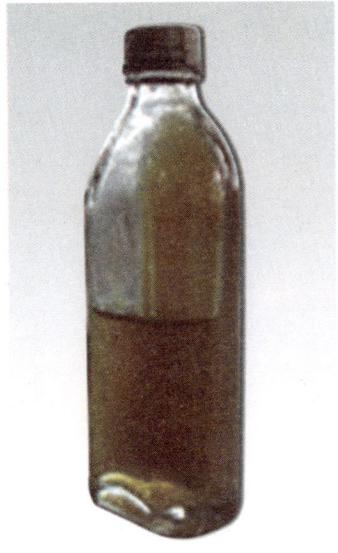

Biphasic fungal blood culture media

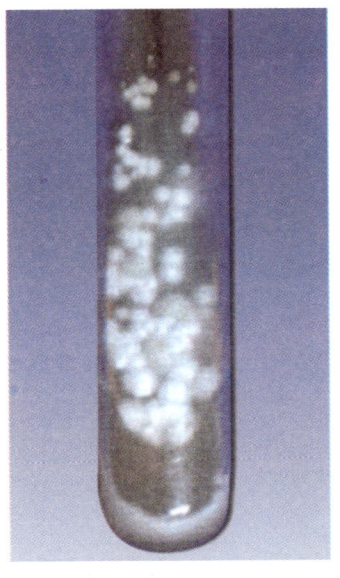

SDA with smooth white creamy growth of yeast

Sabouraud's Dextrose Agar (SDA)

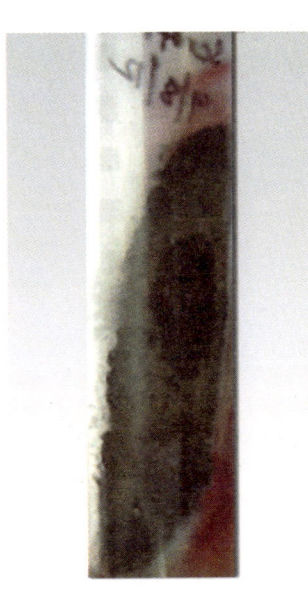

SDA with cottony/woolly/velvety growth of mycelial fungi

Signature of Teacher

Section

5

Entomology Practical

33. Arthropods of Medical Importance

ENTOMOLOGY

Phylum: Arthropoda
Class: Insecta, Arachnida, Crustacae

Characteristics	Class Insecta	Class Arachnida	Class Crustaceae
Body divided into	Head Thorax Abdomen	Cephalothorax Abdomen	Cephalothorax Abdomen
Legs	3 pairs	**Ticks:** Adult—4 pairs Larvae—3 pairs **Mites:** Egg and larva—3 pairs Nymph and adult—4 pairs	5 pairs
Antenna	1 pair	Absent	2 pairs

Wings	**Absent:** Lice, flea, bug
	Present:
	1 pair—mosquito,
	    sandfly,
	    housefly,
	    tsetse fly,
	2 pairs—cockroach,
	    reduviid bug
		Absent	Absent

Examples	Mosquito, fly, lice, flea, bug	Ticks and mites	Cyclops, diaptomus crab, cray fish, fairy shrimps

ENTOMOLOGY

DISEASES TRANSMITTED BY CLASS INSECTA

Mosquito-borne diseases	
Anopheles	Malaria; Chittor virus
Culex	Filariasis; Japanese encephalitis; West Nile fever; sindbis virus
Aedes	Dengue; chikungunya; yellow fever; viral hemorrhagic fever
Mansonoidas	Filariasis
Fly-borne diseases	
Sandfly	Leishmaniasis; sandfly fever; bartonellosis; oriental sore
Tsetse fly (Glossina)	African trypanosomiasis (sleeping sickness)
Housefly (*Musca* spp.)	Mechanical carrier of diarrhoea; dysentry; typhoid fever; trachoma; conjunctivitis; anthrax; yaws; myiasis
Lice-borne diseases	
Head louse (*P. capitis*)	Epidemic typhus; mechanical irritation, dermatitis
Body louse (*P. corporis*)	Epidemic typhus; trench fever; relapsing fever
Pubic louse (*Phthirus pubic*)	No disease India
Flea borne diseases	
Rat flea (*Xenopsylla cheopis*)	Plague; endemic typhus; murine typhus; cestode infection due to *H. diminuta*
Bug-borne diseases	
Cone nosed bugs (reduviid bugs)	Chagas disease (American trypanosomiasis)

ENTOMOLOGY

DISEASES TRANSMITTED BY CLASS ARACHNIDA

	Ticks-borne diseases
Hard tick (ixodid tick) *Dermacentor* spp., *Rhipicephalus* spp. *Haemaphysalis, Ixodes, Ambylomma*	Relapsing fever; tularemia; babesiosis; Lyme disease; Rocky mountain spotted fever; viral encephalitis (KFD) viral hemorrhagic fever; RSSE
Soft tick—Argasidae	Relapsing fever, KFD
	Mite-borne diseases
Scrub mite—trombiculid	Scrub typhus
Itch mite (*Sarcoptes* scabie)	Scabies
Dust mite	Allergy
Rat mite	Rickettsialpox

DISEASES TRANSMITTED BY CLASS CRUSTACEAE (WATER FLEA)

	Crustaceae-borne diseases
Small crustaceans (cyclops, diaptomus)	Dracunculosis, *D. latum* infection
Big crustaceans (crab, cray fish, fairy shrimps)	Transmitting the metacercariae of *P. westermani* (lung fluke)

Arthropods of Medical Importance

Aim: To study characteristic features of various insects/vectors and deseases transmitted to man.

1. *Anopheles* mosquito
2. *Aedes* mosquito
3. Mosquito larvae
4. Housefly
5. Tsetse fly
6. Sandfly
7. Cyclops
8. Hard tick
9. Soft tick
10. Rat flea
11. Itch mite
12. Louse

Characteristic Features of Adult *Anopheles* Mosquito

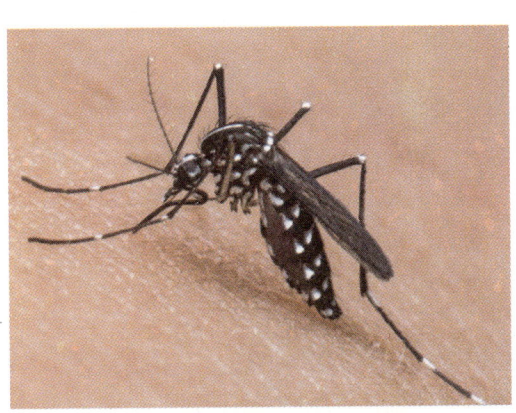

Adult *Anopheles* mosquito

- Adult sits at an angle.
- Wings are spotted at the periphery.
- Diseases transmitted—malaria, Chittoor virus.

Characteristic Features of Adult *Aedes* Mosquito

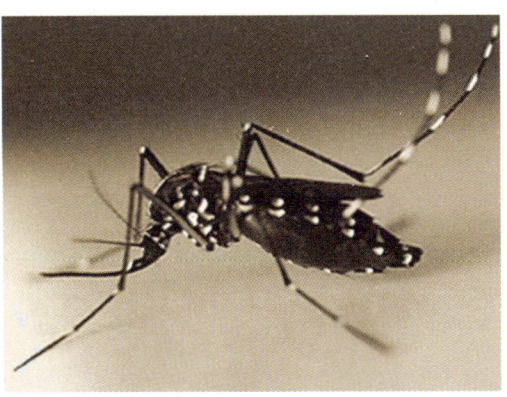

- Black and white stripes on its body and legs
- Bites during day time
- Breeds in clean stagnant water

Adult *Aedes* mosquito

Mosquito Larvae

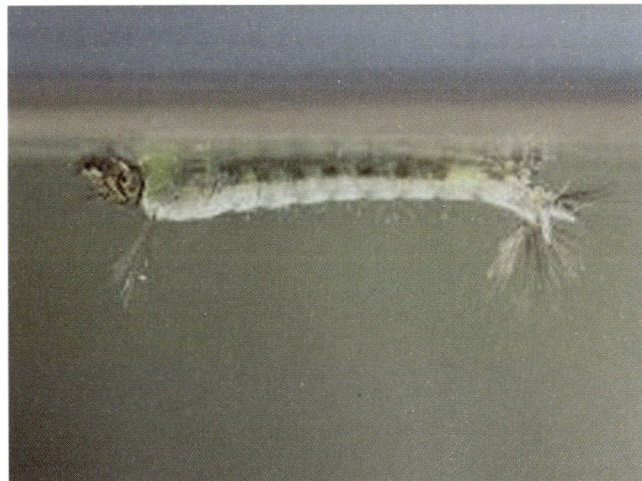

Anopheles larva

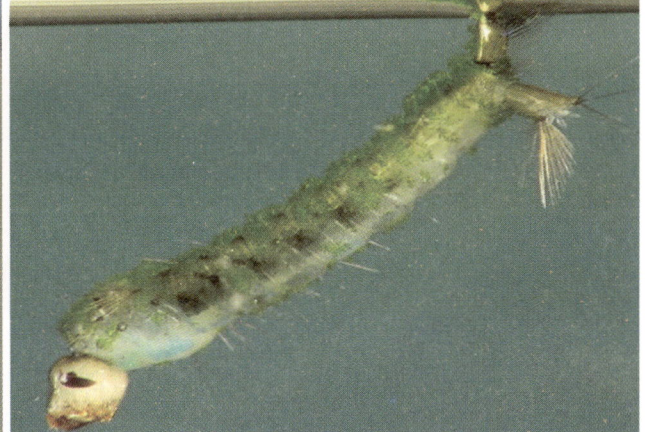

Aedes larva

Characteristic Features of Housefly

- A pair of antennae, short retractile proboscis, compound eye
- Thorax bears a pair of wings and three pairs of hairy legs
- Act as mechanical transmitters of diseases like enteric fever, gastroenteritis causing agents, trachoma, myiasis, etc.

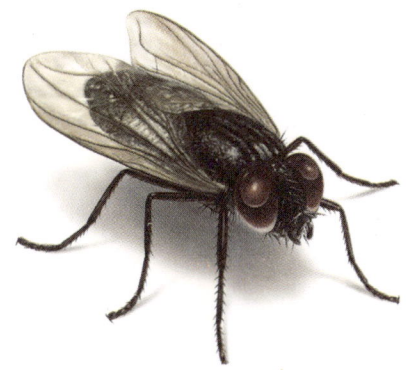

Housefly

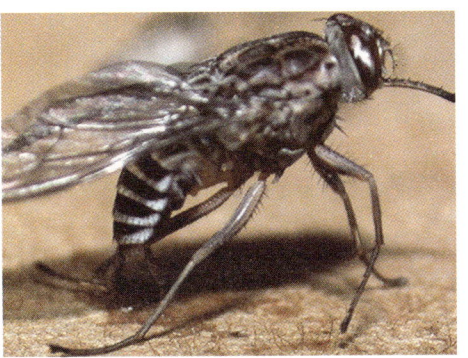

Testse fly

Characteristic Features of Tsetse Fly

- Yellow or dark brown—resembles housefly
- Wings when folded overlap each other like blades of scissors
- Rigid, non-retractile proboscis adapted for skin piercing
- Disease transmitted trypanosomiasis—"sleeping sickness"

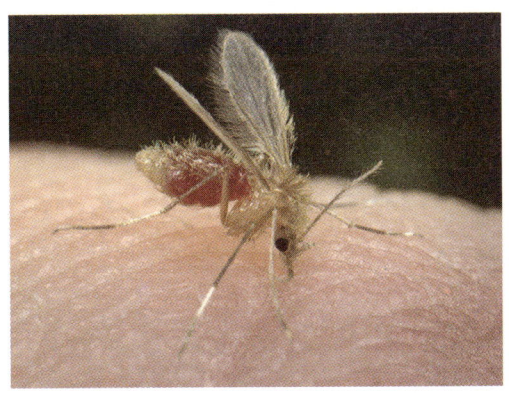

Sandfly

Characteristic Features of Sandfly

- Small insect 1.5–2 mm in length—body and wings densely haired
- Long slender and hairy antennae, palpi and proboscis
- Thorax bears a pair of wings and three pairs of legs
- Wings are upright and lanceolate, hairy—second longitudinal vein branches twice with first branching at the middle of the wing—characteristic of the genus *Phlebotomus*
- Legs are long and slender and out of proportion to the body
- Sandflies hop and do not fly

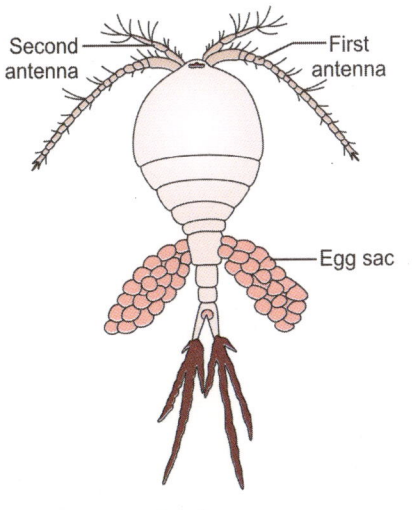

Cyclops

Characteristics Features of Cyclops

- Not more than 1 mm in length
- Pear-shaped semi-transparent body
- Forked tail
- 2 pairs of antennae
- 5 pairs of legs
- A small pigmented eye
- Transmits dracunculiasis and fish tapeworm (*Diphyllobothrium latum*) infestation

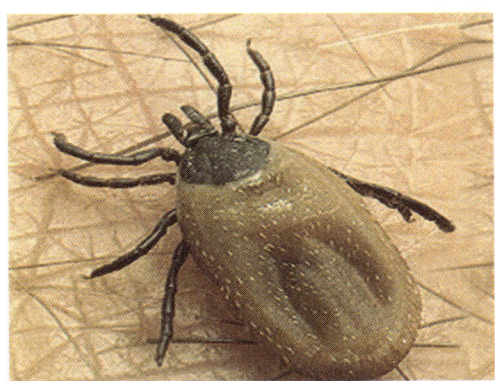

Hard tick

Characteristics Features of Hard Tick

- Scutum present—entire in males, small portion in front in females
- Head anterior
- Several hundred or thousand eggs laid at one sitting
- Cannot starve—bites day and night
- Diseases transmitted: Babesious, tularemia, tick typhus Lyme disease

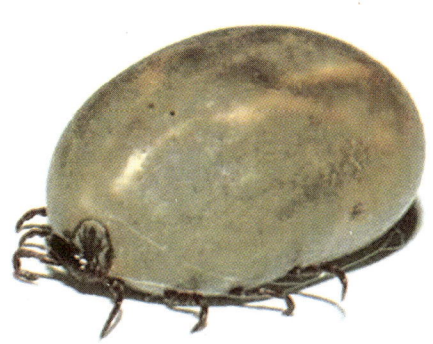

Soft tick

Characteristic Features of Soft Tick

- Scutum absent
- Head ventral—not seen from above
- Laid in batches 20–100 over a long period of time
- Can starve for a year or more
- Diseases transmitted—borreliasis, relapsing fever, Q-fever, KFD

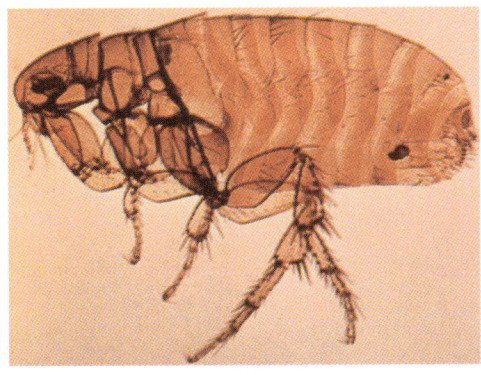

Rat flea

Characteristic Features of Rat Flea

- The insect is laterally flattened.
- Conical head without a neck—piercing mouth parts project downwards and are conspicuous
- Three segmented thorax—pro-, meso- and meta-thorax—no wings
- Three pairs of strong legs
- 10 segmented abdomen—males have a coiled structure—the penis; females have a short, stumpy structure—the spermatheca
- **Cannot fly—jumps** vertically 4 inches when starved or 3 inches when fed and can jump horizontally up to 6 inches
- Diseases transmitted: Endemic typhus and bubonic plague.

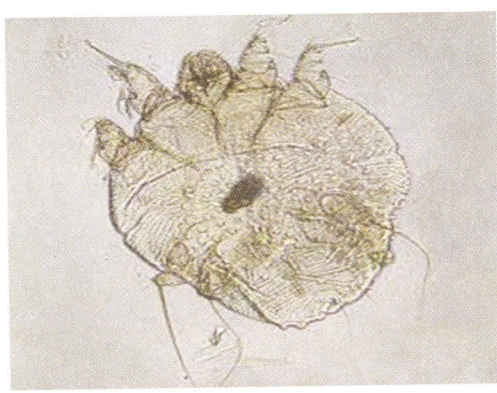

Itch mite

Characteristic Features of Itch Mite

- 0.4 mm size
- **Body:** No demarcation between cephalothorax and abdomen.
  - 2 pairs of legs in front—suckers
  - 2 pairs of legs behind—long bristle
- Male has sucker in all the legs except the 3rd pair which distinguishes it from female.
- Disease transmitted: Scabies

Characteristic Features of Louse

- Head is pointed in front, 5 jointed antennae, mouth parts adapted for sucking blood
- Thorax fused mass, square-shaped
- Strongly built three pairs of legs with claws
- 9-segmented elongated abdomen
- **Diseases transmitted:**
  - Epidemic typhus
  - Relapsing fever (epidemic)
  - Trench fever
  - Dermatitis
- **Species:**
  - Head louse—*Pediculus capitis*
  - Body louse—*Pediculus corporis*
  - Pubic or crab louse—*Phthirus pubis*

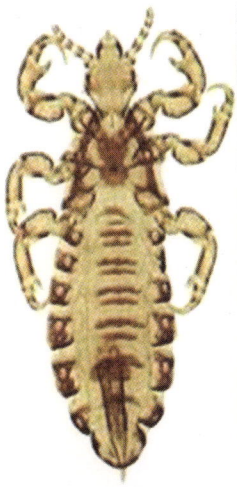

Head louse   **Body louse**

Signature of Teacher

6

Virology Practical

34. Virology Methods

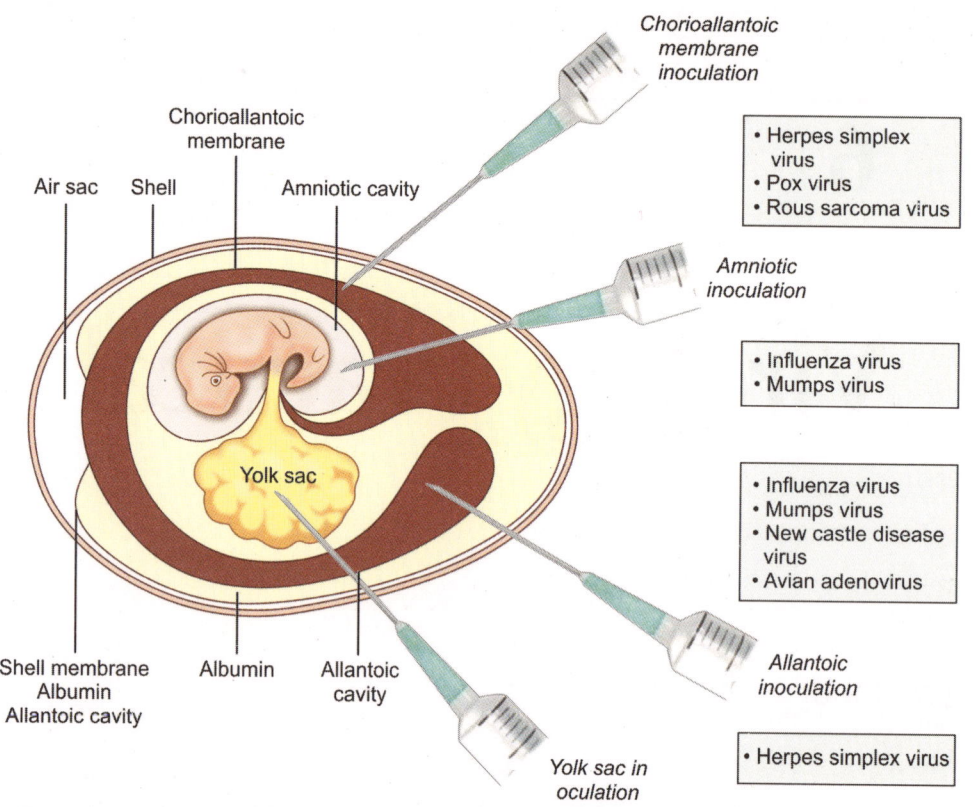

• Herpes simplex
  virus
• Pox virus
• Rous sarcoma virus

• Influenza virus
• Mumps virus

• Influenza virus
• Mumps virus
• New castle disease
  virus
• Avian adenovirus

• Herpes simplex virus

Growth of viruses in embryonated hen's EGG
An embryonated hen's egg showing the different compartments in which viruses may grow.
The different routes by which viruses are inoculated into eggs are indicated.

Virology Methods

Aim: To study the different routes of inoculation for isolation of viruses from embryonated hen's egg and different methods for diagnosis of viruses.

Demonstration

1. Tissue culture bottle
2. Viral transport medium
3. Microtitre plate
4. Methods of inoculation of embryonated eggs
5. Hemagglutination test
6. Multinucleated giant cells of HSV
7. Negri body

Microtitre Plate

- It is a flat plate with multiple "wells" (96 wells).
- Made of polystyrene, polypropylene or polycarbonate.
- Wells have either a conical/flat/round bottom.
- Uses:
  – ELISA for diagnosis of HIV, HBV, HCV.
  – Hemagglutination test
  – Hemagglutination inhibition test
  – Complement fixation.
  – TPHA test (*Treponema pallidum* hemagglutination)

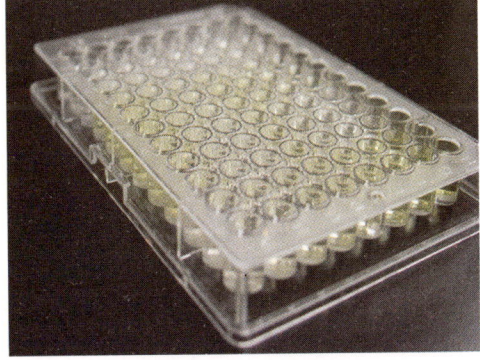

Microtitre plate

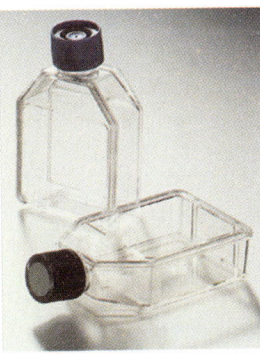

Tissue culture bottles

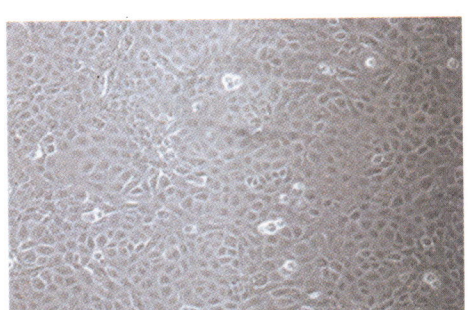

A monolayer of vero cell (verbet monkey kidney cell, continuous cell line)

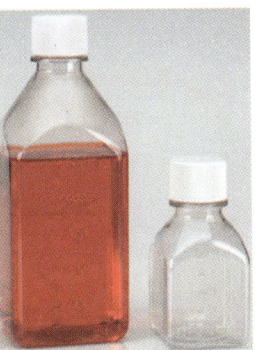

Viral transport medium (pink to red)

155

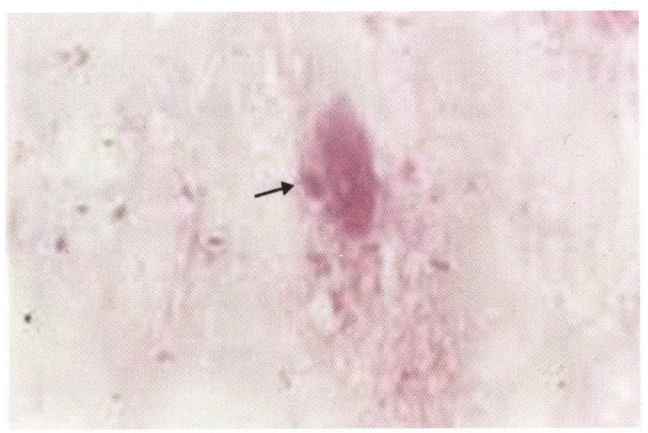

Impression smear from hippocampus of a rabid dog showing magenta colored intracellular Negri body (arrow) in a neuron. Seller's stain

Negri Body

- Specific intra-cytoplasmic eosinophillic inclusion body found in the cytoplasm of large neurons (1–10/cell) in rabies
- 2–20μm, sharply defined, spherical/oval/elongated
- Cherry red to magenta colored, uniformly stained
- Larger Negri bodies contain blue staining granules/inner bodies, often arranged in concentric layers
- Part of the brain that best demonstrates Negri bodies is the Ammon horn of hippocampus
- Stain used: Seller stain
- Negri bodies are found in infection with street virus but not fixed virus
- Sensitivity of Negri bodies in rabies is 65–68%.

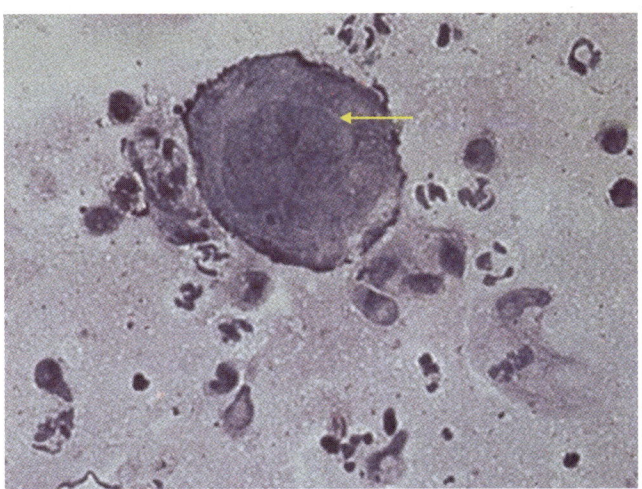

Giemsa stained Tzank smear from genital ulcer showing multinucleated giant cells of HSV-2

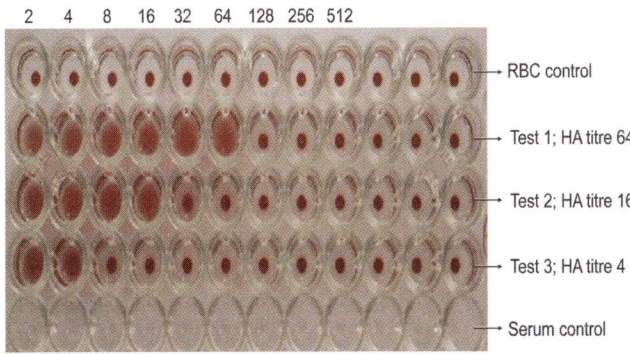

Hemagglutination test

Signature of Teacher